PALEO
SMOOTHIES AND JUICES

pil

Publications International, Ltd.

Pictured on the front cover: Blackberry Lime Smoothie *(page 102)*.

Pictured on the back cover *(left to right):* Berry Mojito Smoothie (page 144), Tangy Apple Kale Smoothie (page 62) and Sunset Berry (page 204).

ISBN: 978-1-68022-701-7

Library of Congress Control Number: 2016945923

Manufactured in China.

8 7 6 5 4 3 2 1

TABLE OF CONTENTS

BREAKFAST BLENDS

JUST PEACHY CANTALOUPE SMOOTHIE
MAKES 2 SERVINGS

- ¼ cup orange juice
- 2 cups frozen sliced peaches
- 1½ cups cantaloupe chunks
- 1 tablespoon almond butter

Combine orange juice, peaches, cantaloupe and almond butter in blender; blend until smooth.

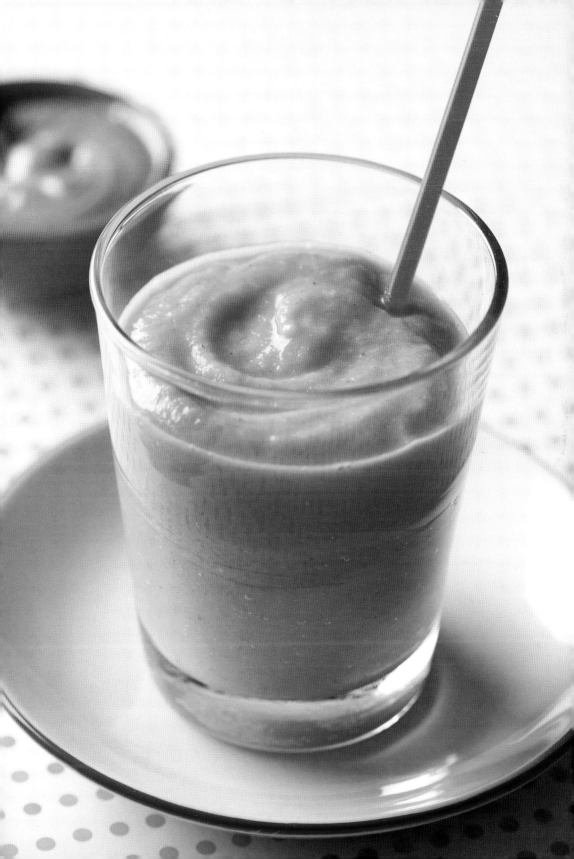

BANANA CHAI SMOOTHIE
MAKES 2 SERVINGS

¾ cup water

¼ cup unsweetened coconut milk

2 frozen bananas

1 teaspoon honey

¼ teaspoon ground ginger

¼ teaspoon ground cinnamon

¼ teaspoon vanilla

Pinch ground cloves (optional)

Combine water, coconut milk, bananas, honey, ginger, cinnamon, vanilla and cloves, if desired, in blender; blend until smooth.

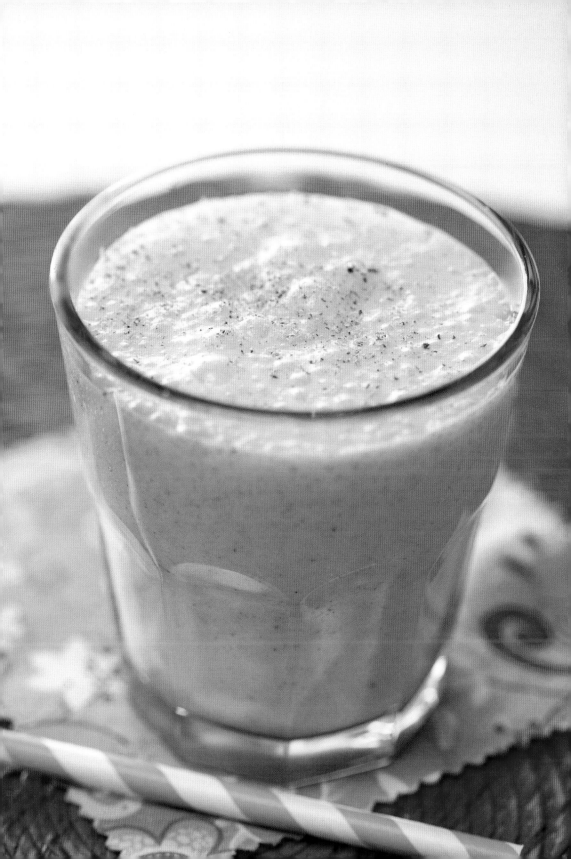

MANGO CITRUS SMOOTHIE
MAKES 2 SERVINGS

2 tangerines

1 cup frozen mango chunks

¼ cup ice cubes

Juice of 1 lime

1 tablespoon honey

1 Grate peel from tangerines; peel and seed tangerines.

2 Combine tangerine sections and grated peel in blender with mango, ice, lime juice and honey; blend until smooth.

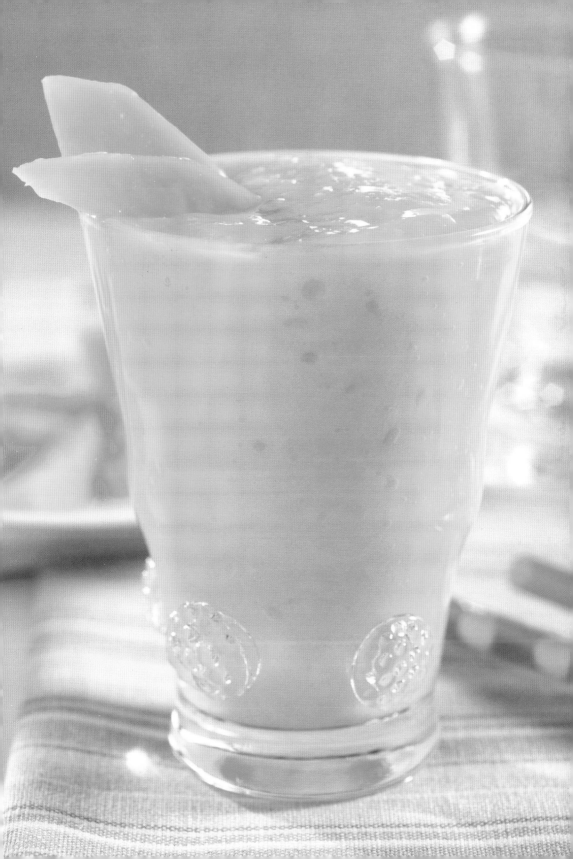

CANTALOUPE STRAWBERRY SUNRISE >

MAKES 2 SERVINGS

- **1 cup cantaloupe chunks**
- **2 clementines, peeled**
- **1 cup frozen strawberries**

Combine cantaloupe, clementines and strawberries in blender; blend until smooth.

HONEYDEW GINGER SMOOTHIE

MAKES 1 SERVING

- **1 cup honeydew chunks**
- **½ cup frozen banana slices**
- **2 tablespoons water**
- **½ teaspoon grated fresh ginger**

Combine honeydew, banana, water and ginger in blender; blend until smooth.

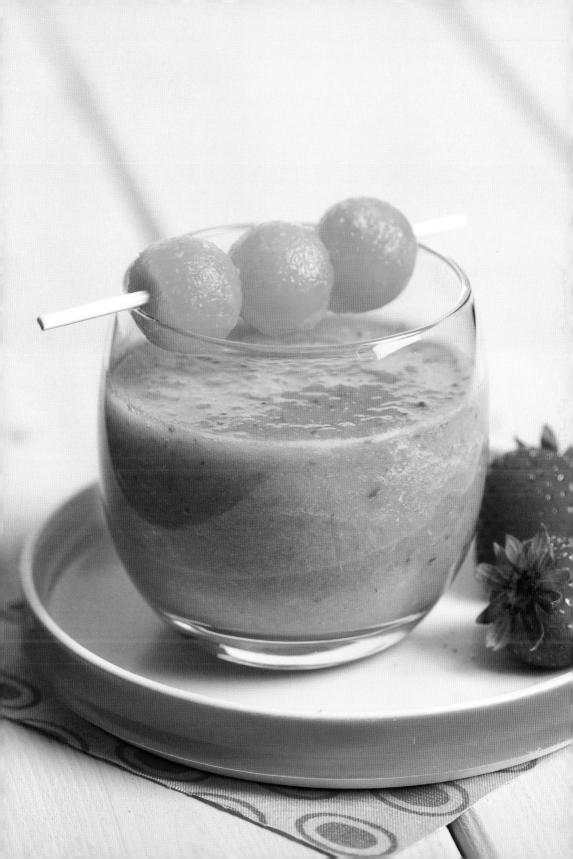

QUADRUPLE ORANGE SMOOTHIE
MAKES 2 SERVINGS

½ **cup water**

3 **carrots, peeled and cut into chunks**

1 **navel orange, peeled and seeded**

1 **clementine, peeled**

½ **cup frozen mango chunks**

Combine water, carrots, orange, clementine and mango in blender; blend until smooth.

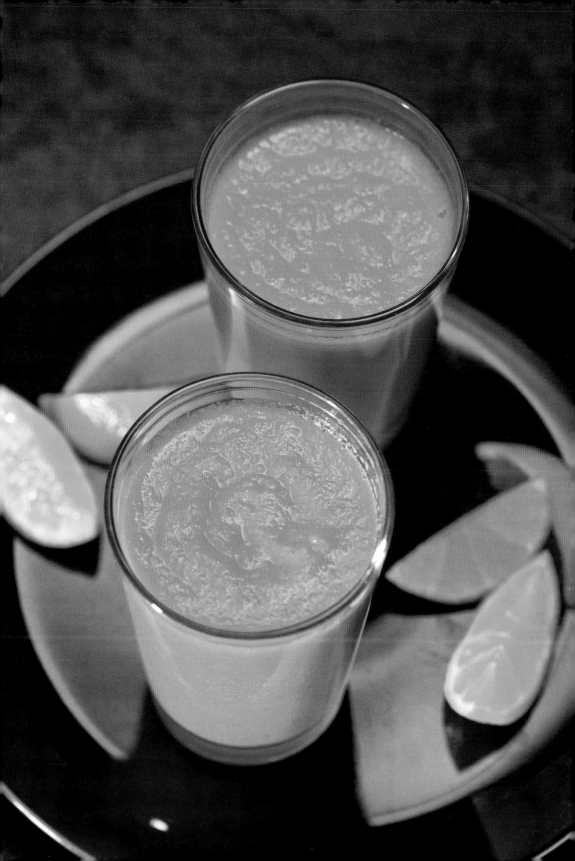

BREAKFAST POM SMOOTHIE
MAKES 2 SERVINGS

¾ cup pomegranate juice

½ cup unsweetened almond milk

1 frozen banana

½ cup sliced fresh strawberries

½ cup fresh blueberries

Combine pomegranate juice, almond milk, banana, strawberries and blueberries in blender; blend until smooth.

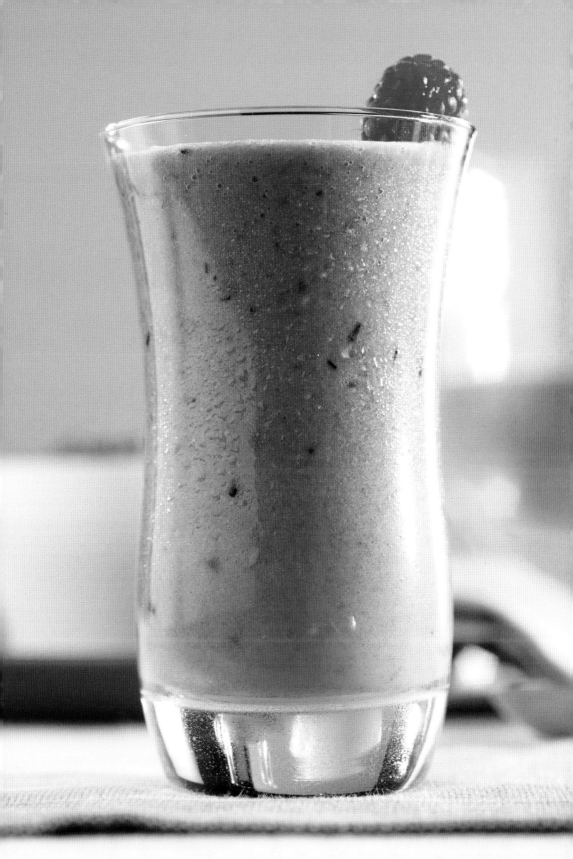

CREAMY STRAWBERRY-BANANA SHAKE

MAKES 3 SERVINGS

¾ cup orange juice

2¼ cups ice cubes

1 banana

¾ cup fresh strawberries, hulled

½ avocado, pitted and peeled

Combine orange juice, ice, banana, strawberries and avocado in blender; blend until smooth.

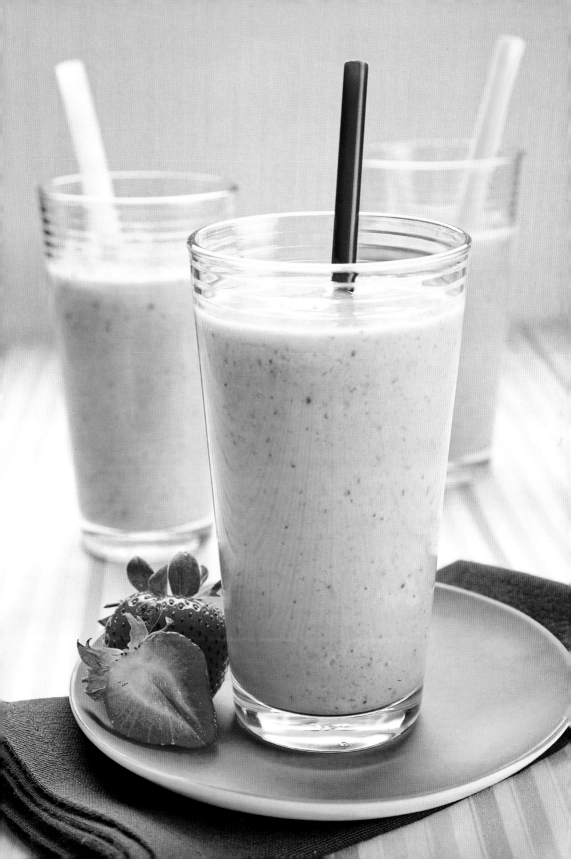

MANGO MADNESS
MAKES 2 SERVINGS

½ cup unsweetened almond milk

¼ cup water

¼ cup orange juice

1 cup frozen mango chunks

½ cup frozen sliced peaches

½ banana

Combine almond milk, water, orange juice, mango, peaches and banana in blender; blend until smooth.

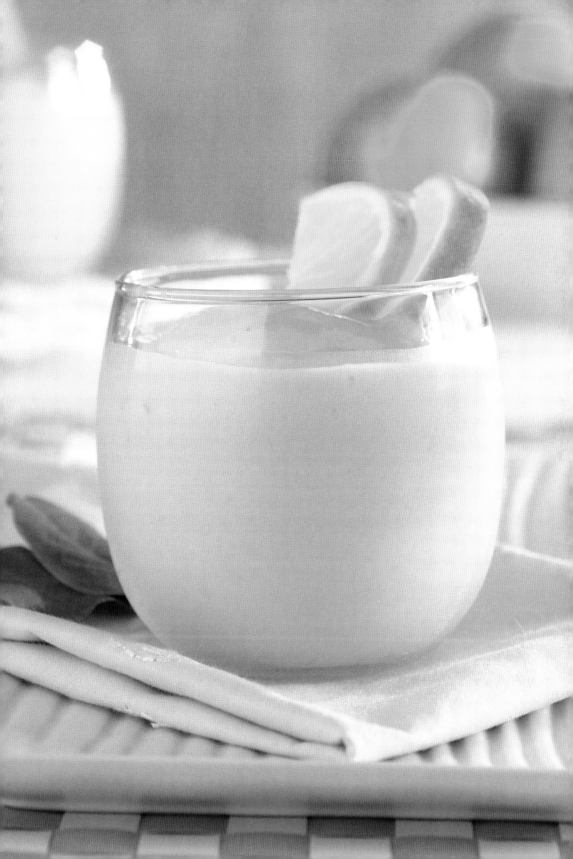

CREAMY CHOCOLATE SMOOTHIE >
MAKES 1 SERVING

1 cup unsweetened almond milk

1 frozen banana

½ avocado, pitted and peeled

1 tablespoon honey

1 tablespoon unsweetened cocoa powder

Combine almond milk, banana, avocado, honey and cocoa in blender; blend until smooth.

TROPICAL BREAKFAST SMOOTHIE
MAKES 2 SERVINGS

¼ cup orange juice

1 cup fresh pineapple chunks

½ banana

¼ cup ice cubes

2 tablespoons flaked coconut

½ tablespoon lime juice

Combine orange juice, pineapple, banana, ice, coconut and lime juice in blender; blend until smooth.

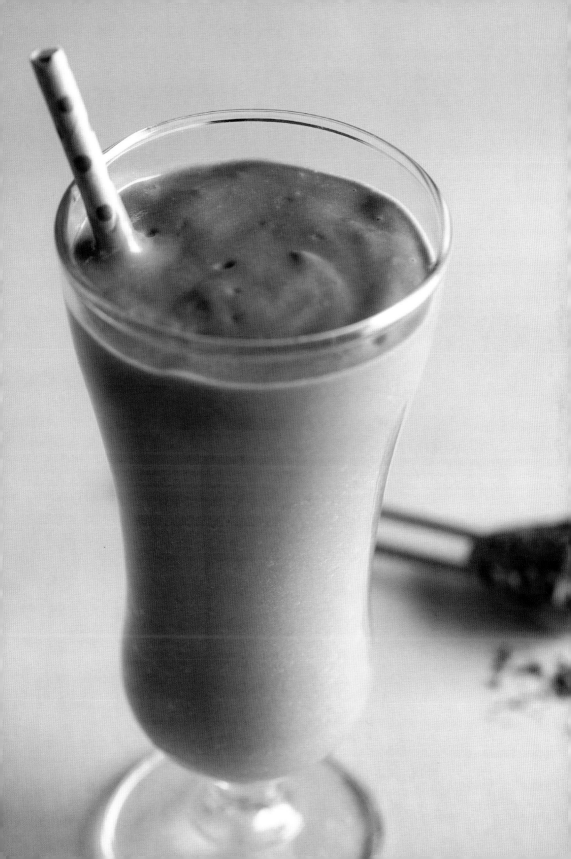

MORNING GLORY SMOOTHIE
MAKES 2 SERVINGS

1 pink or ruby red grapefruit, peeled and seeded

1 banana

¾ cup frozen strawberries

1 teaspoon honey

Combine grapefruit, banana, strawberries and honey in blender; blend until smooth.

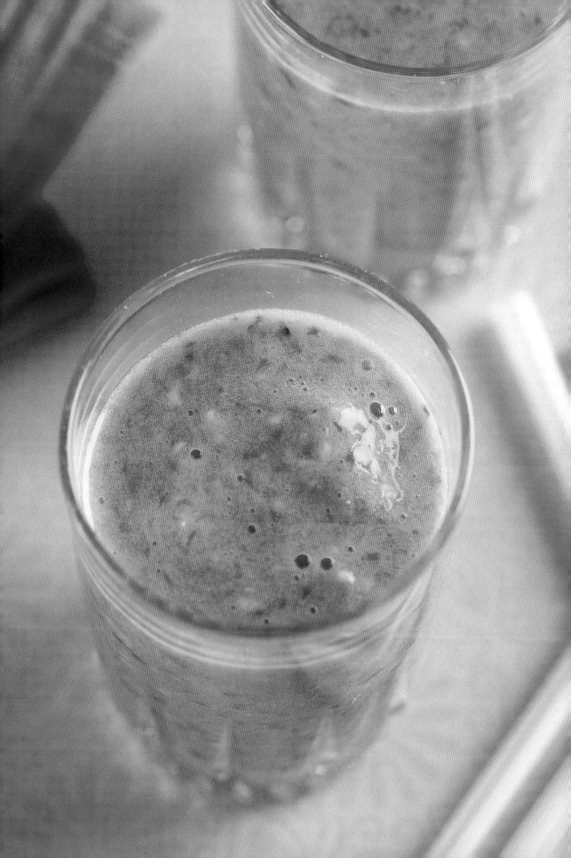

BANANA-PINEAPPLE BREAKFAST SHAKE

MAKES 2 SERVINGS

- ½ cup unsweetened almond milk
- 1 cup fresh pineapple chunks
- 1 frozen banana
- ½ cup ice cubes
- 1 teaspoon vanilla
- ⅛ teaspoon ground nutmeg

Combine almond milk, pineapple, banana, ice, vanilla and nutmeg in blender; blend until smooth.

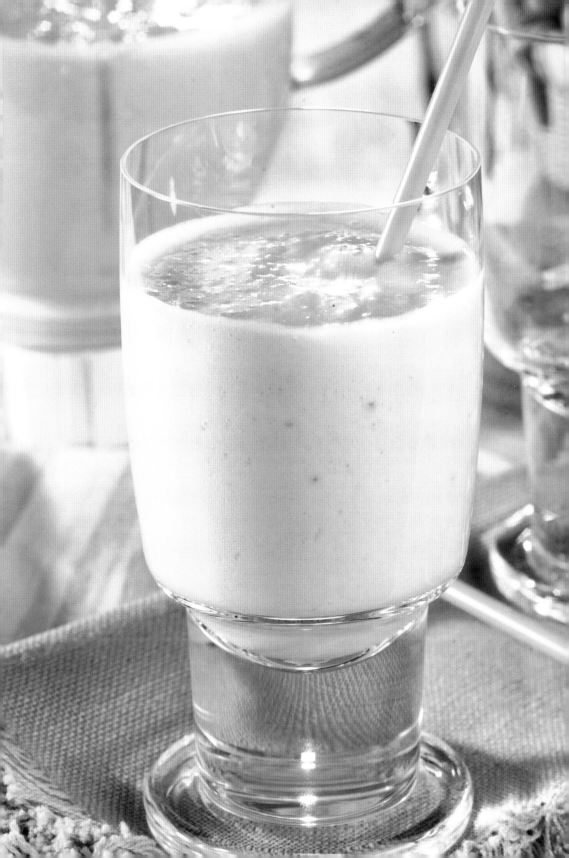

STRAWBERRY MANGO SMOOTHIE

MAKES 3 SERVINGS

¾ cup apricot juice

2 cups fresh strawberries, hulled

1 cup frozen mango chunks

¼ cup ice cubes

Combine apricot juice, strawberries, mango and ice in blender; blend until smooth.

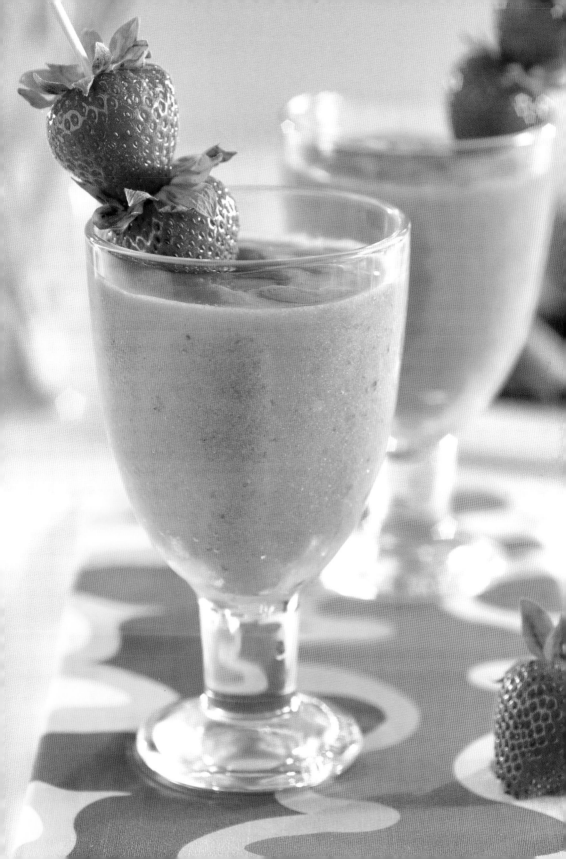

FRUIT FAVORITES

ORCHARD MEDLEY
MAKES 3 SERVINGS

½ cup water

2 plums, pitted and cut into chunks

1 sweet red apple, seeded and cut into chunks

1 pear, seeded and cut into chunks

2 teaspoons lemon juice

Combine water, plums, apple, pear and lemon juice in blender; blend until smooth.

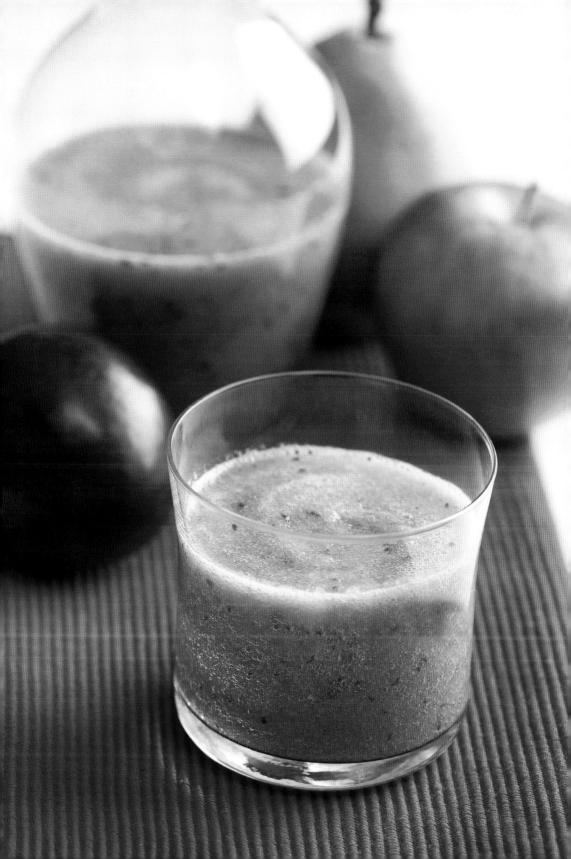

RUBY RED DELIGHT
MAKES 2 SERVINGS

¼ **cup water**

1 **navel orange, peeled and seeded**

1 **medium beet, peeled and cut into chunks**

½ **cup seedless red grapes**

½ **cup frozen strawberries**

¼ **teaspoon ground ginger**

Combine water, orange, beet, grapes, strawberries and ginger in blender; blend until smooth.

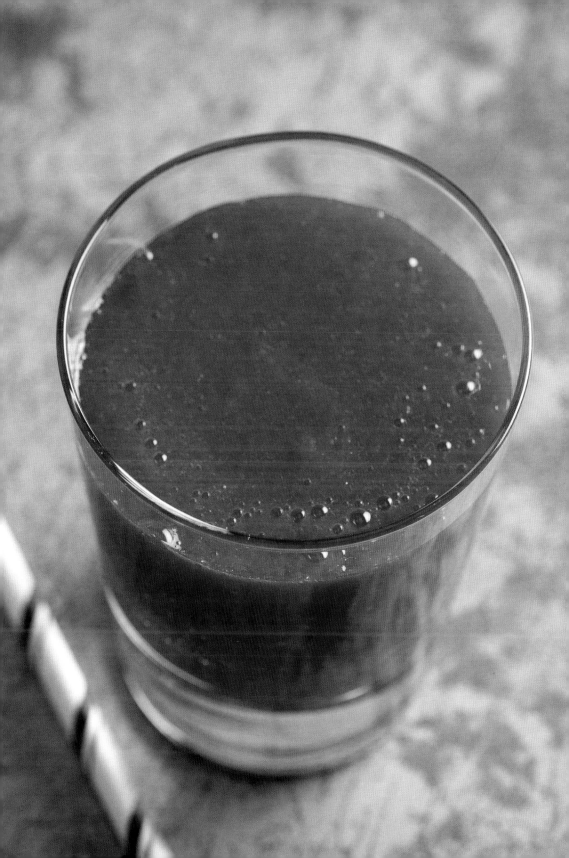

CARROT CAKE SMOOTHIE
MAKES 1 SERVING

½ **cup coconut water**

3 **carrots, peeled and cut into chunks**

½ **banana**

½ **cup frozen pineapple chunks**

1 **teaspoon honey**

⅛ **teaspoon ground cinnamon**

⅛ **teaspoon ground ginger**

Combine coconut water, carrots, banana, pineapple, honey, cinnamon and ginger in blender; blend until smooth.

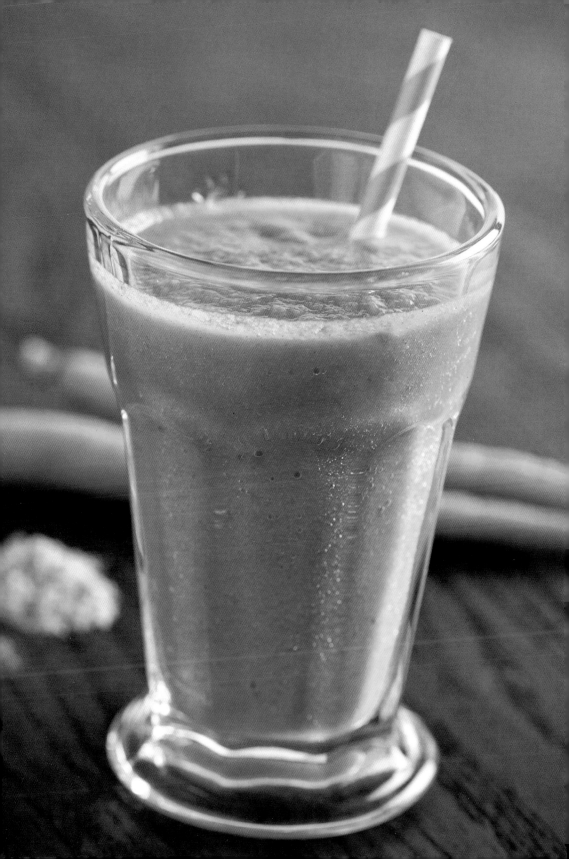

CANTALOUPE SMOOTHIE >

- ½ **orange juice**
- 2 **cups cantaloupe chunks**
- ½ **cup ice cubes**
- ½ **teaspoon vanilla**

Combine orange juice, cantaloupe, ice and vanilla in blender; blend until smooth.

TANGERAPPLE SMOOTHIE

MAKES 1 SERVING

- 1 **sweet red apple, seeded and cut into chunks**
- 1 **tangerine, peeled and seeded**
- 1 **frozen banana**

Combine apple, tangerine and banana in blender; blend until smooth.

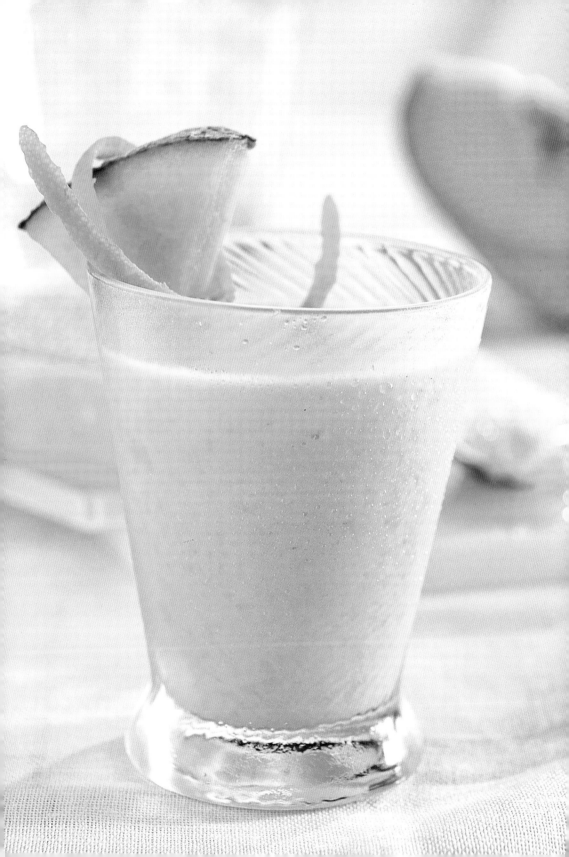

GREAT GRAPE ESCAPE
MAKES 2 SERVINGS

¼ cup water

1 tangerine, peeled and seeded

1 cup frozen seedless red grapes

½ cup frozen raspberries

1 teaspoon lemon juice

Combine water, tangerine, grapes, raspberries and lemon juice in blender; blend until smooth.

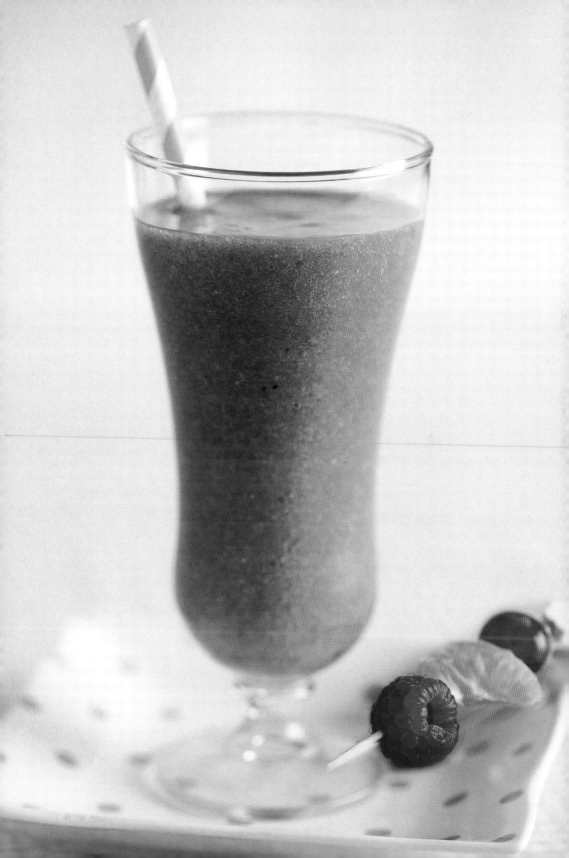

CHERRY COOLER
MAKES 3 SERVINGS

- 3 cups orange juice
- 8 ounces fresh cherries, pitted
- ½ teaspoon vanilla
- ½ cup ice cubes

Combine orange juice, cherries, vanilla and ice in blender; blend until smooth.

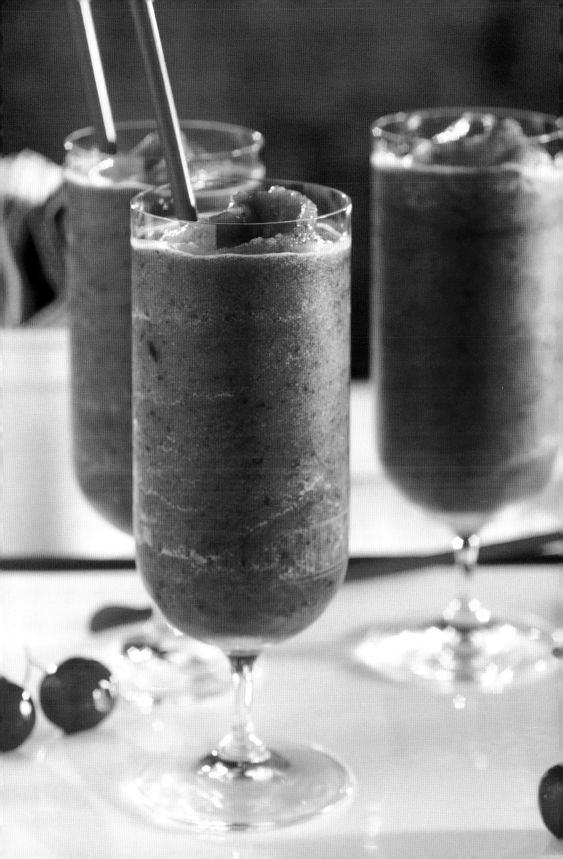

SWEET SPINACH SENSATION
MAKES 2 SERVINGS

½ **cup water**

1 **sweet red apple, seeded and cut into chunks**

1 **tangerine, peeled and seeded**

1 **cup frozen mango chunks**

1 **cup baby spinach**

Combine water, apple, tangerine, mango and spinach in blender; blend until smooth.

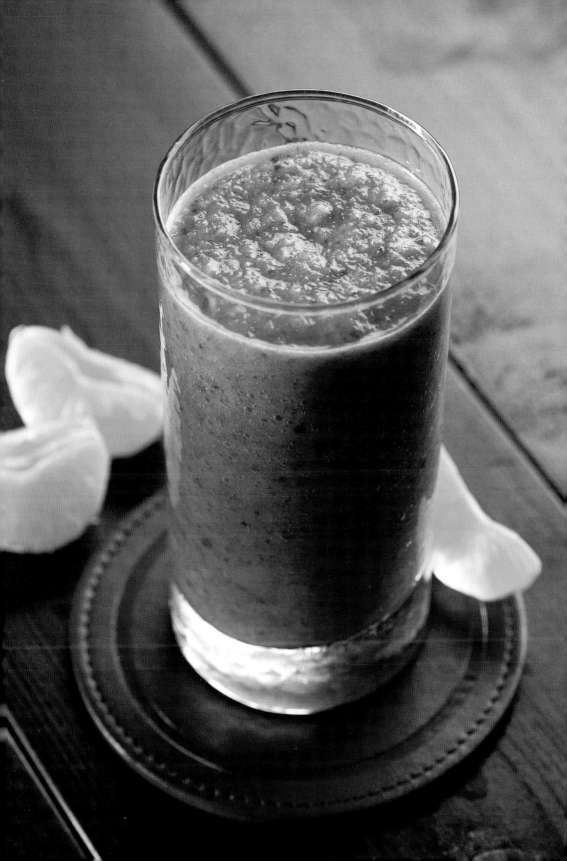

KIWI STRAWBERRY SMOOTHIE >
MAKES 3 SERVINGS

1½ cups unsweetened coconut milk

3 kiwis, peeled and quartered

1½ cups sliced fresh strawberries

¾ cup ice cubes

1½ tablespoons honey

Combine coconut milk, kiwis, strawberries, ice and honey in blender; blend until smooth.

EASY APPLE PIE SMOOTHIE
MAKES 1 SERVING

½ cup water

1 sweet red apple, seeded and cut into chunks

1 tablespoon honey

¼ teaspoon ground cinnamon

¼ teaspoon vanilla

Pinch *each* ground allspice and ground nutmeg

Combine water, apple, honey, cinnamon, vanilla, allspice and nutmeg in blender; blend until smooth.

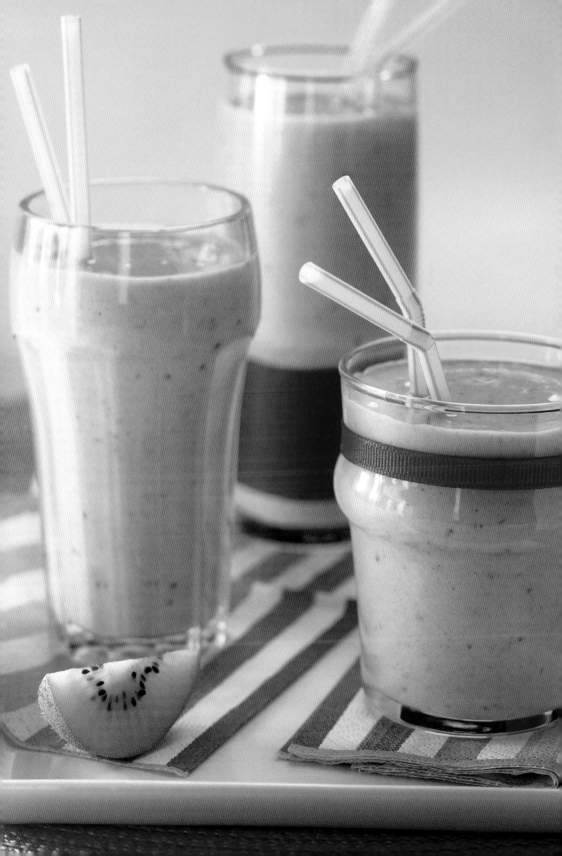

PURPLE PLEASER SMOOTHIE
MAKES 3 SERVINGS

½ cup water

2 cups seedless red grapes

2 cups frozen blackberries

2 cups baby spinach

½ cup ice cubes

¼ teaspoon ground cinnamon

Combine water, grapes, blackberries, spinach, ice and cinnamon in blender; blend until smooth.

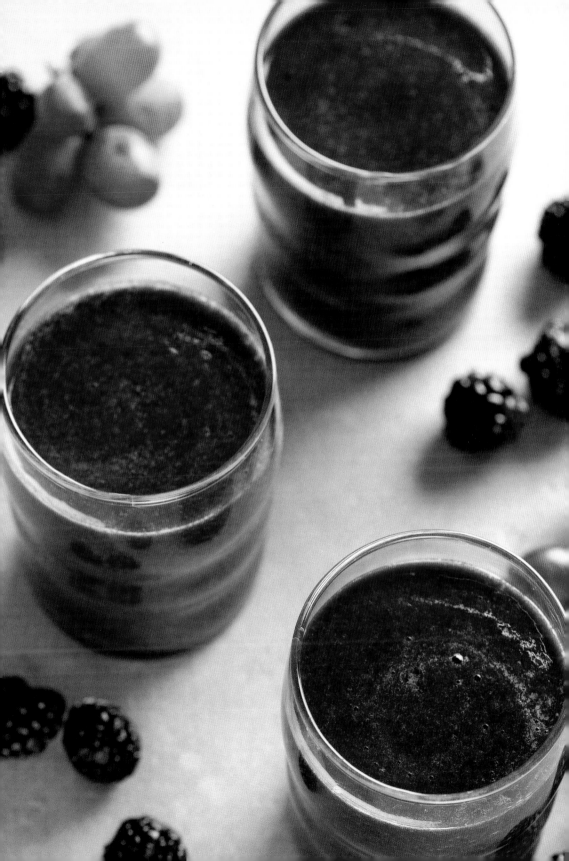

PEACH APRICOT PARADISE
MAKES 2 SERVINGS

½ **cup dried apricots**

¼ **cup water**

¼ **cup orange juice**

 1 **cup frozen sliced peaches**

¼ **teaspoon ground ginger**

1 Place apricots in small bowl; cover with hot water. Let stand 10 minutes or until soft; drain.

2 Combine ¼ cup water, orange juice, peaches, apricots and ginger in blender; blend until smooth.

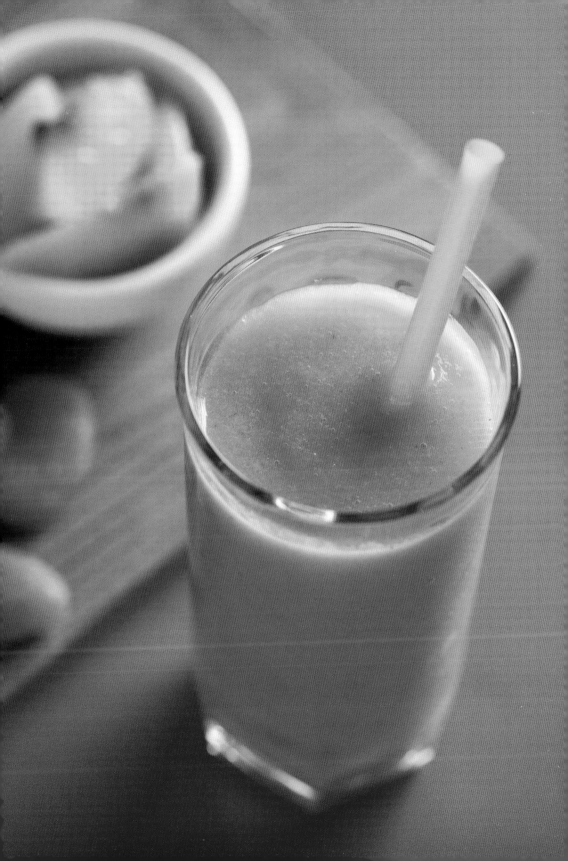

STRAWBERRY APPLE SMOOTHIE
MAKES 2 SERVINGS

¾ cup water

1 sweet red apple, seeded and cut into chunks

1 clementine, peeled

1 cup frozen strawberries

1 tablespoon lemon juice

Combine water, apple, clementine, strawberries and lemon juice in blender; blend until smooth.

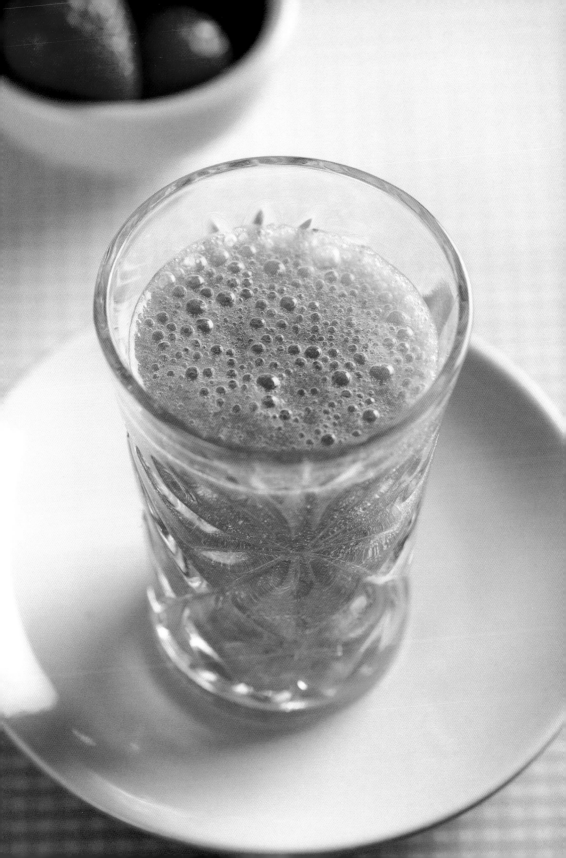

GOING GREEN

TRIPLE GREEN SMOOTHIE
MAKES 2 SERVINGS

2 cups seedless green grapes

1 kiwi, peeled and quartered

½ avocado, pitted and peeled

Combine grapes, kiwi and avocado in blender; blend until smooth.

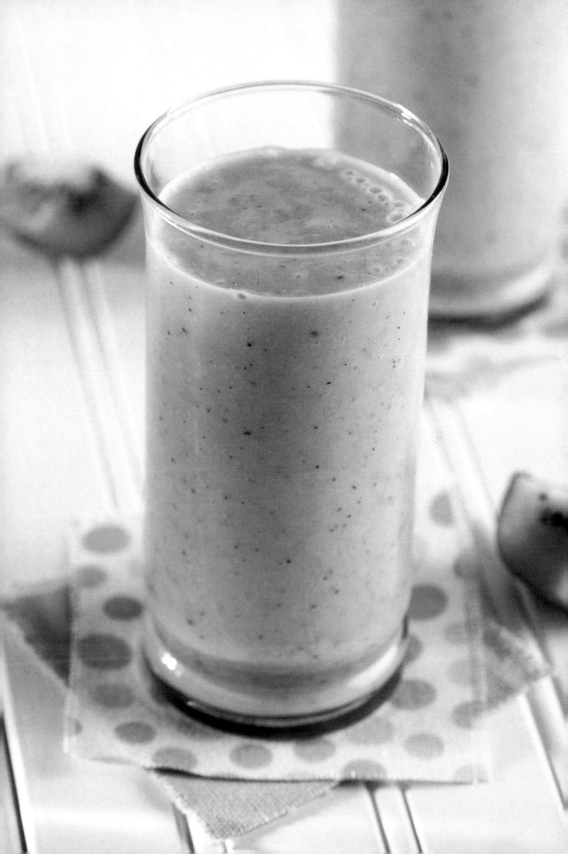

SPINACH APPLE SATISFACTION
MAKES 1 SERVING

¼ cup apple juice

1 Granny Smith apple, seeded and cut into chunks

1 cup baby spinach

½ cup ice cubes

½ avocado, pitted and peeled

1 teaspoon almond butter

½ teaspoon grated fresh ginger

Combine apple juice, apple, spinach, ice, avocado, almond butter and ginger in blender; blend until smooth.

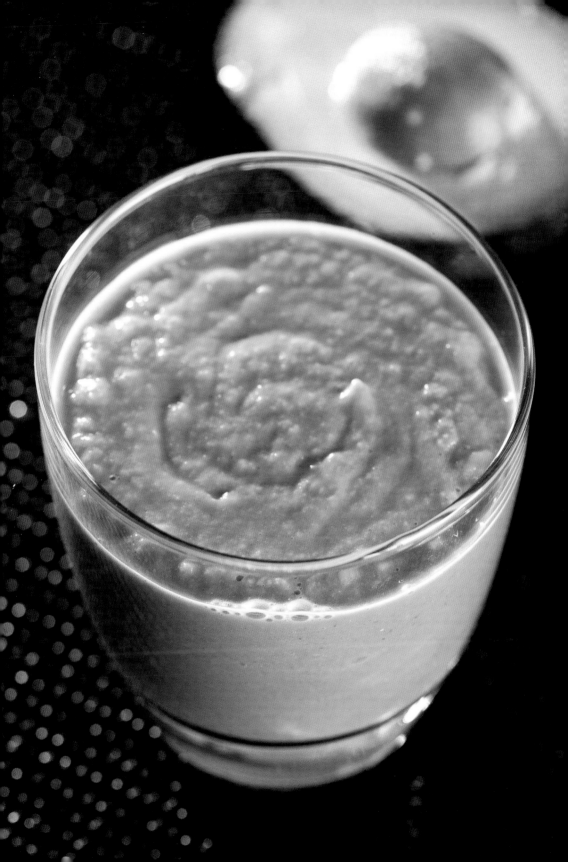

TROPICAL GREEN SHAKE
MAKES 3 SERVINGS

¾ **cup orange juice**

1½ **cups packed stemmed kale**

1½ **cups frozen tropical fruit mix***

1½ **cups ice cubes**

3 **tablespoons honey**

Tropical mix typically contains pineapple, mango and strawberries along with other fruit.

Combine orange juice, kale, tropical fruit mix, ice and honey in blender; blend until smooth.

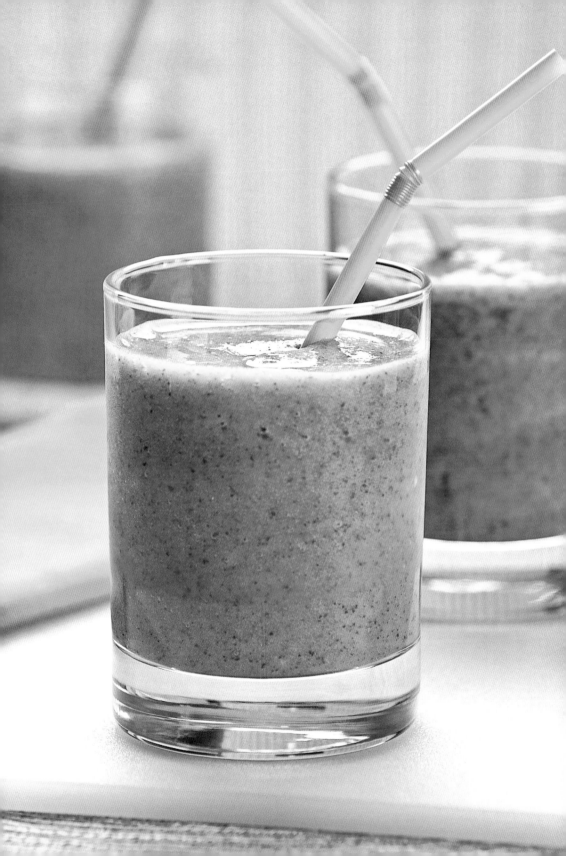

SWEET GREEN SUPREME

MAKES 2 SERVINGS

2 cups seedless green grapes

½ cup ice cubes

½ frozen banana

½ cup baby kale

Combine grapes, ice, banana and kale in blender; blend until smooth.

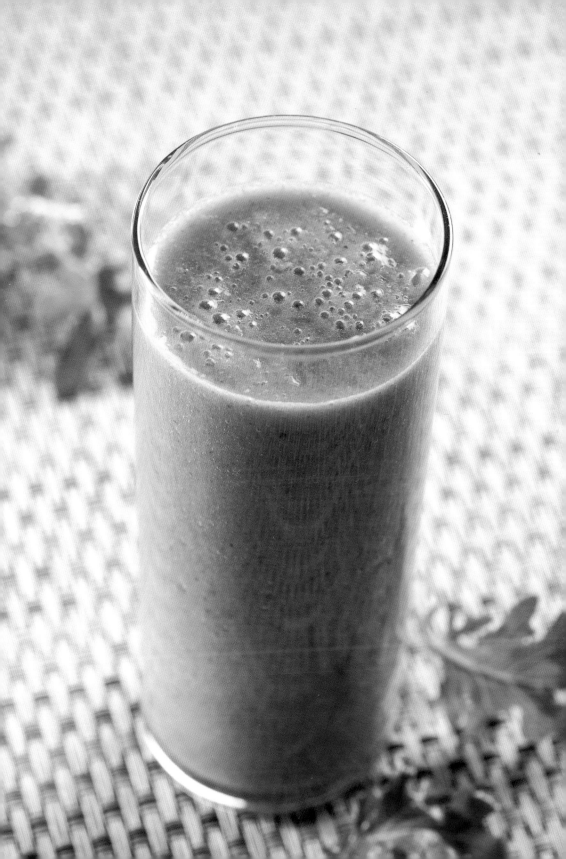

CHERRY GREEN SMOOTHIE
MAKES 2 SERVINGS

1 cup unsweetened almond milk

1½ cups frozen dark sweet cherries

¾ cup baby spinach

½ frozen banana

1 tablespoon ground flaxseed

2 teaspoons honey

Combine almond milk, cherries, spinach, banana, flaxseed and honey in blender; blend until smooth.

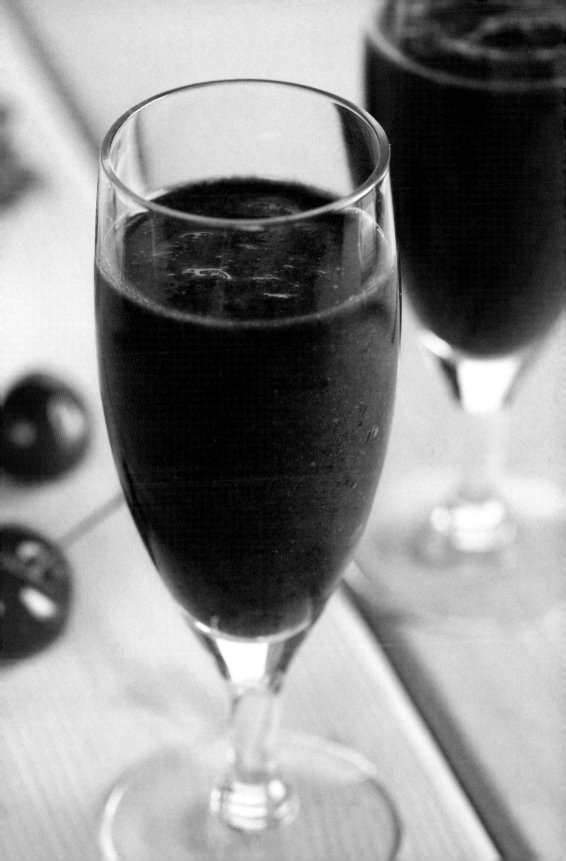

GO GREEN SMOOTHIE

MAKES 2 SERVINGS

½ cup unsweetened almond milk

2 cups baby spinach

1 cup seedless green grapes

1 avocado, pitted and peeled

1 cup ice cubes

2 teaspoons honey

Combine almond milk, spinach, grapes, avocado, ice and honey in blender; blend until smooth.

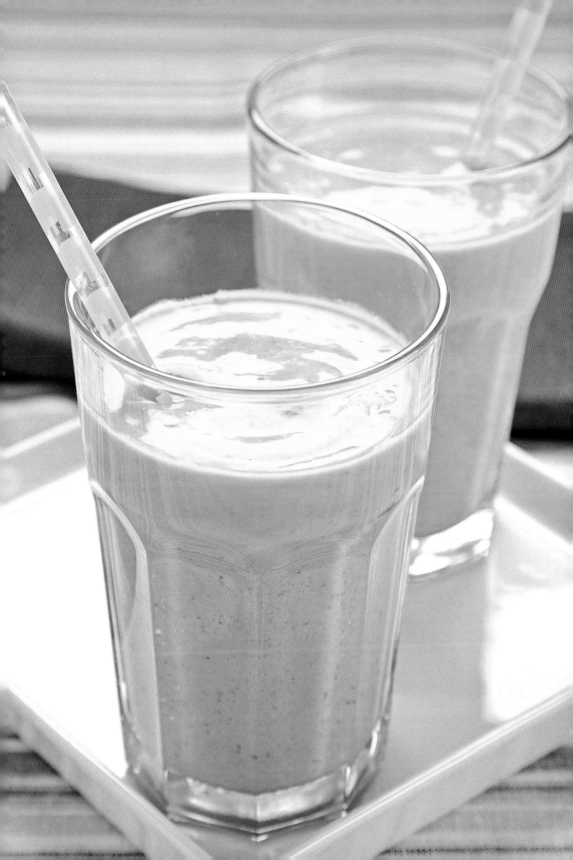

TANGY APPLE KALE SMOOTHIE >
MAKES 3 SERVINGS

1 cup water

2 Granny Smith apples, seeded and cut into chunks

2 cups baby kale

1 frozen banana

Combine water, apples, kale and banana in blender; blend until smooth.

PEAR AVOCADO SMOOTHIE
MAKES 2 SERVINGS

1 cup apple juice

1½ cups ice cubes

1 pear, seeded and cut into chunks

½ avocado, pitted and peeled

½ cup fresh mint

2 tablespoons lime juice

Combine apple juice, ice, pear, avocado, mint and lime juice in blender; blend until smooth.

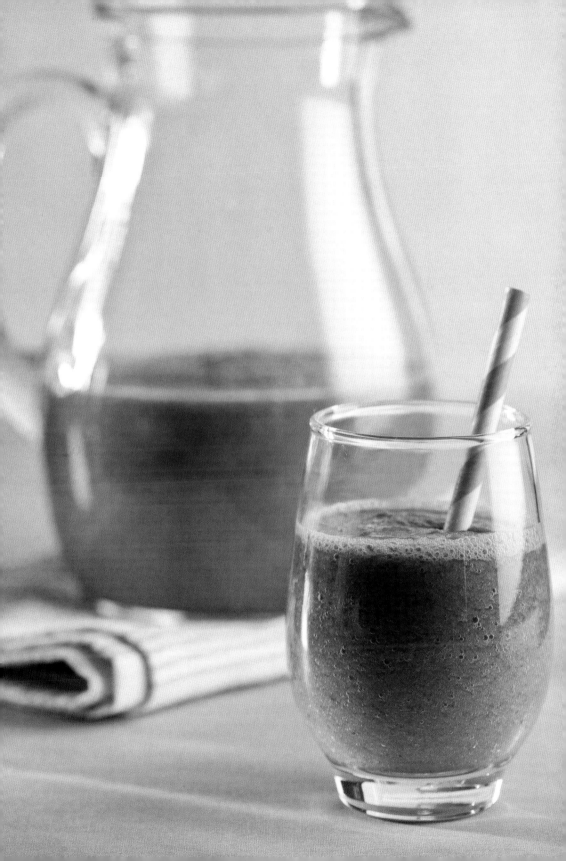

PEACHES AND GREEN
MAKES 1 SERVING

¾ cup unsweetened almond milk

1 cup packed spinach

1 cup frozen sliced peaches

1 cup ice cubes

2 tablespoons honey

½ teaspoon vanilla

Combine almond milk, spinach, peaches, ice, honey and vanilla in blender; blend until smooth.

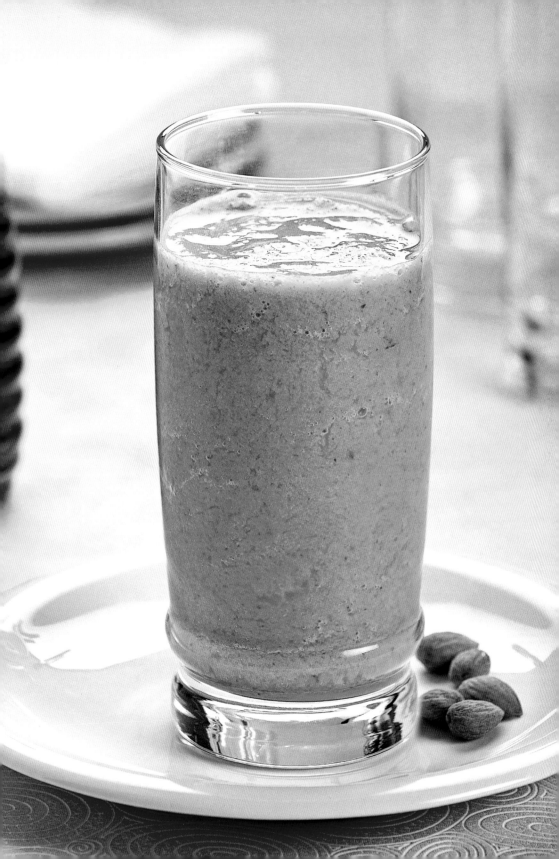

GREEN ISLANDER SMOOTHIE
MAKES 2 SERVINGS

2 cups ice cubes

1 banana

1½ cups fresh pineapple chunks

1 cup packed spinach

1 cup packed stemmed kale

Combine ice, banana, pineapple, spinach and kale in blender; blend until smooth.

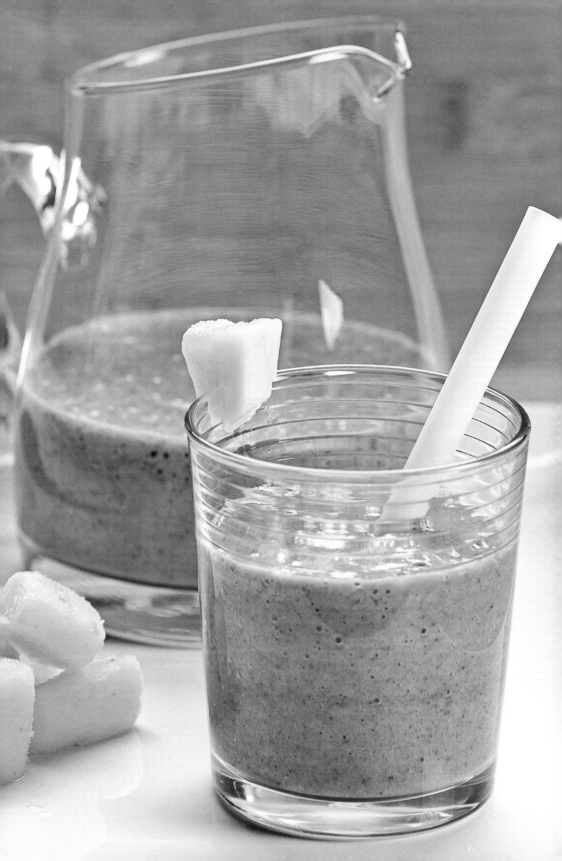

GLORIOUSLY GREEN
MAKES 2 SERVINGS

1 cup ice cubes

1½ cups honeydew chunks

2 kiwis, peeled and quartered

½ cup green seedless grapes

1 tablespoon honey

Combine ice, honeydew, kiwis, grapes and honey in blender; blend until smooth.

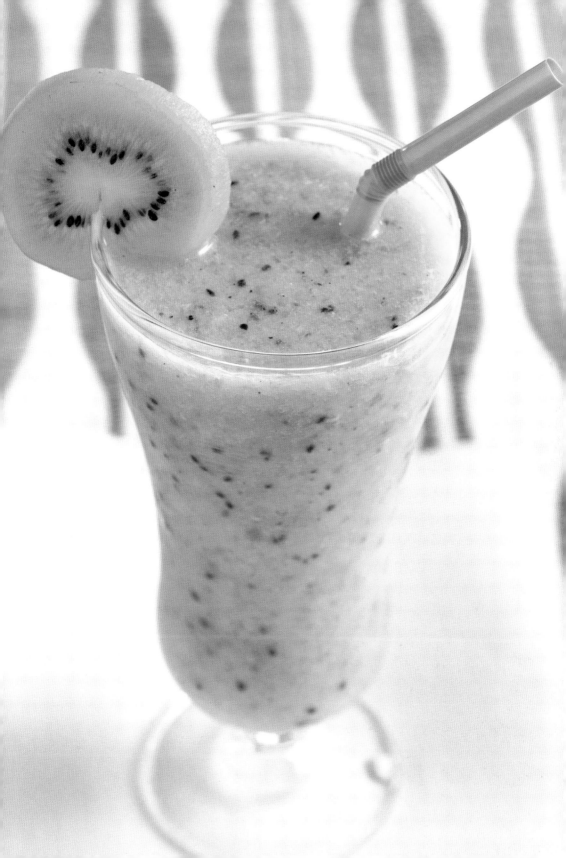

GREENS GALORE
MAKES 2 SERVINGS

¼ cup water

2 small Granny Smith apples, seeded and cut into chunks

1 cup baby spinach

½ cucumber, peeled and cut into chunks

¼ cup ice cubes

⅓ cup fresh mint

Combine water, apples, spinach, cucumber, ice and mint in blender; blend until smooth.

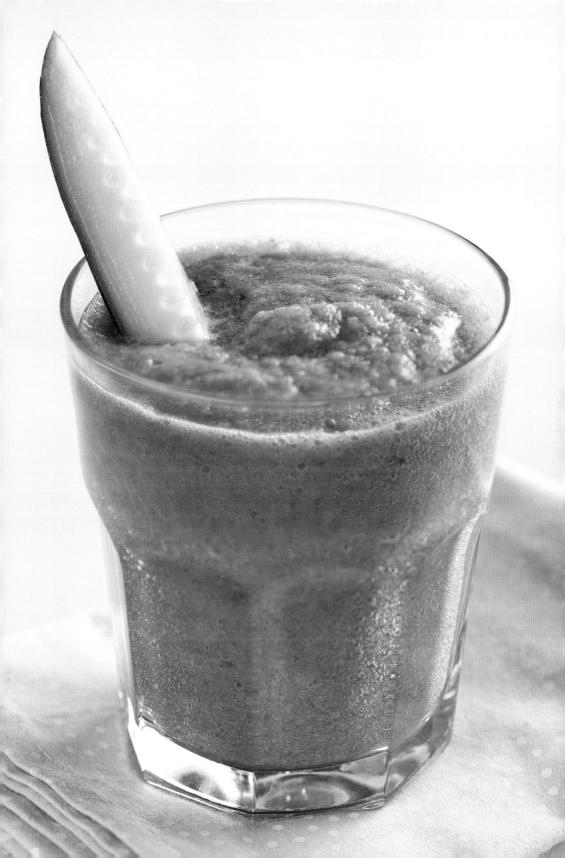

GREEN CANTALOUPE QUENCHER
MAKES 2 SERVINGS

2 cups cantaloupe chunks

1 cup frozen pineapple chunks

1 cup baby spinach

1 tablespoon ground flaxseed

Combine cantaloupe, pineapple, spinach and flaxseed in blender; blend until smooth.

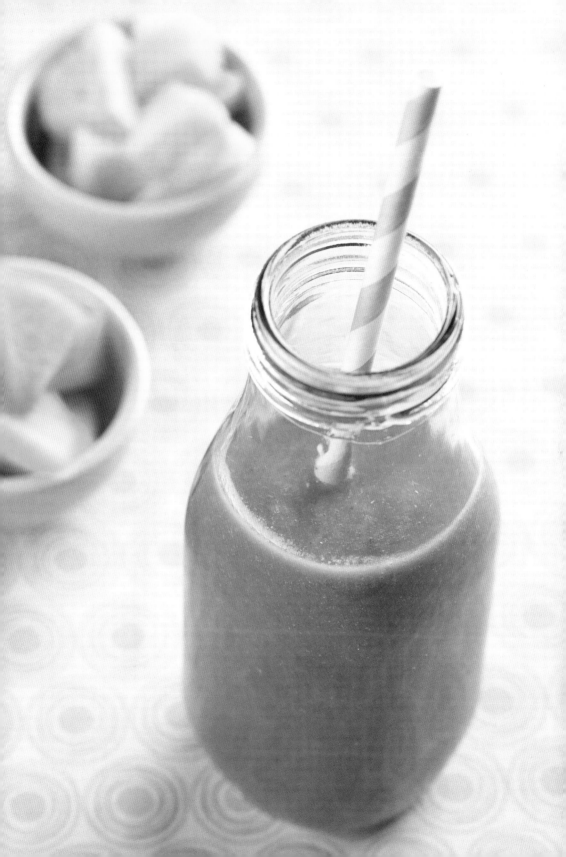

TROPICAL TREATS

TROPICAL STORM SMOOTHIE
MAKES 2 SERVINGS

¼ cup water

1 cup papaya chunks

1 cup frozen pineapple chunks

½ frozen banana

1 tablespoon lemon juice

⅛ teaspoon ground cinnamon

Combine water, papaya, pineapple, banana, lemon juice and cinnamon in blender; blend until smooth.

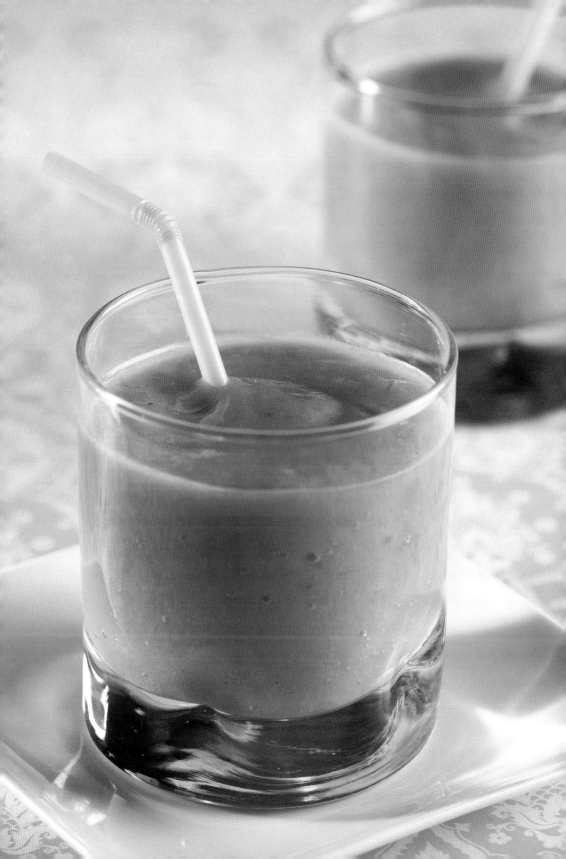

PINEAPPLE CRUSH
MAKES 1 SERVING

- ½ **cup unsweetened coconut milk**
- 1½ **cups frozen pineapple chunks**
- ¼ **cup ice cubes**
- ½ **teaspoon vanilla**

Combine coconut milk, pineapple, ice and vanilla in blender; blend until smooth.

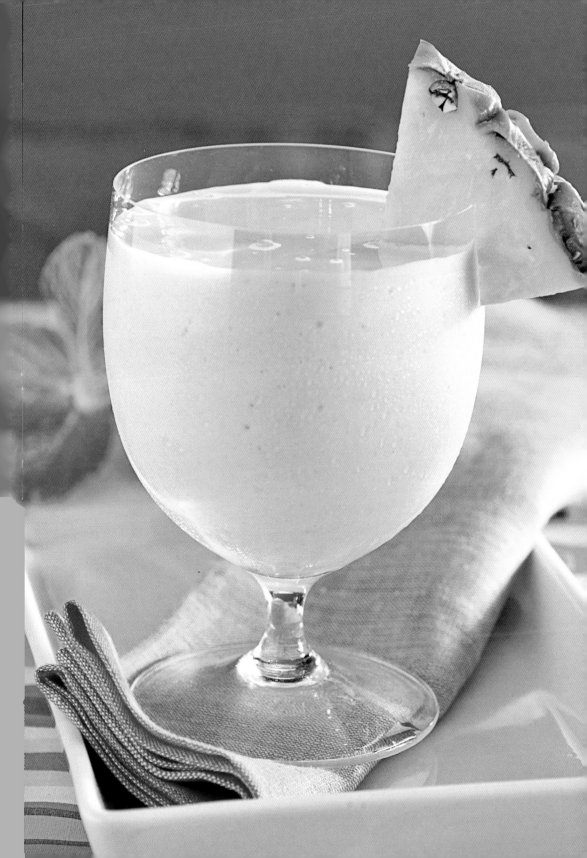

STRAWBERRY BANANA COCONUT SMOOTHIE
MAKES 3 SERVINGS

1¼ cups unsweetened coconut milk

2 cups frozen strawberries

1 banana

¼ cup ice cubes

1 tablespoon honey

Combine coconut milk, strawberries, banana, ice and honey in blender; blend until smooth.

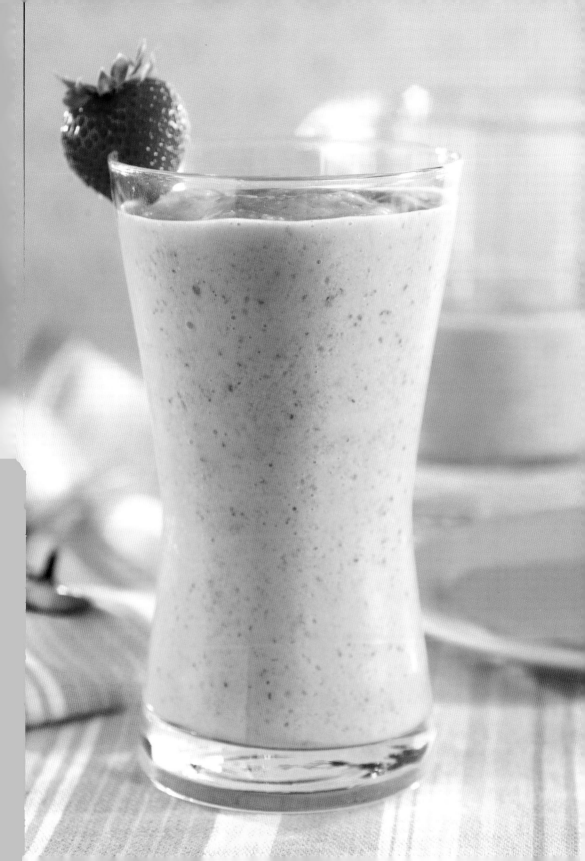

TROPICAL SUNRISE
MAKES 2 SERVINGS

⅓ cup unsweetened coconut milk

⅓ cup orange juice

1 frozen banana

1 cup frozen mango chunks

½ cup fresh pineapple chunks

Combine coconut milk, orange juice, banana, mango and pineapple in blender; blend until smooth.

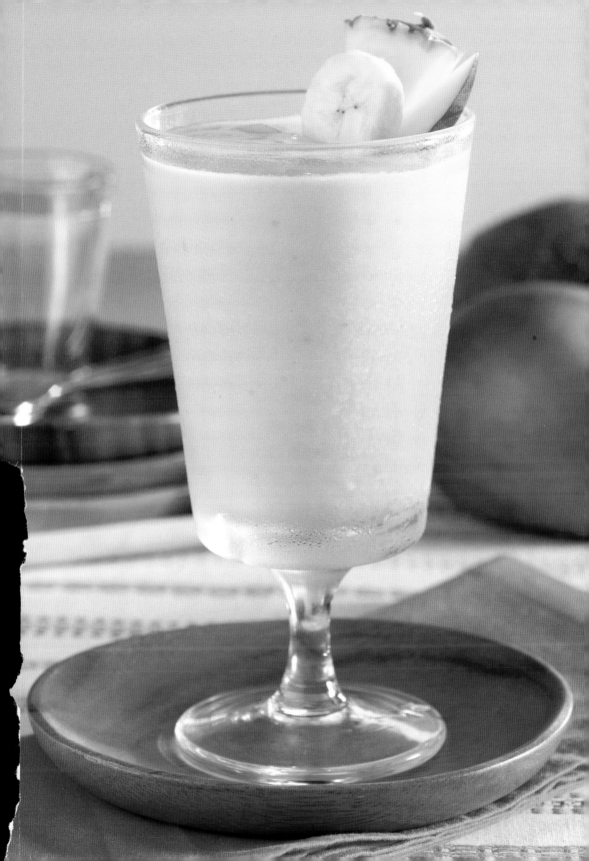

PAPAYA-PINEAPPLE SMOOTHIE >

MAKES 2 SERVINGS

½ cup pineapple juice

2 cups papaya chunks

1 cup frozen pineapple chunks

1 tablespoon lime juice

1 to 2 tablespoons honey*

*Increase honey to 2 tablespoons depending on sweetness of papaya.

Combine pineapple juice, papaya, pineapple, lime juice and honey in blender; blend until smooth.

PIÑA COLADA SMOOTHIE

MAKES 1 SERVING

¾ cup unsweetened coconut milk

¾ cup frozen pineapple chunks

½ banana

Combine coconut milk, pineapple and banana in blender; blend until smooth.

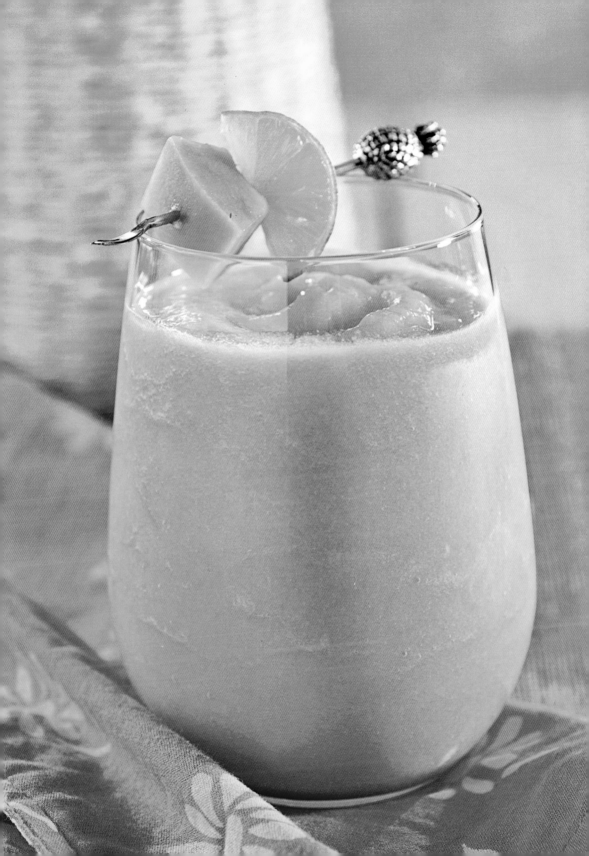

ISLAND DELIGHT SMOOTHIE
MAKES 2 SERVINGS

1 cup unsweetened almond milk

1 frozen banana

½ cup frozen mango chunks

1 tablespoon almond butter

Combine almond milk, banana, mango and almond butter in blender; blend until smooth.

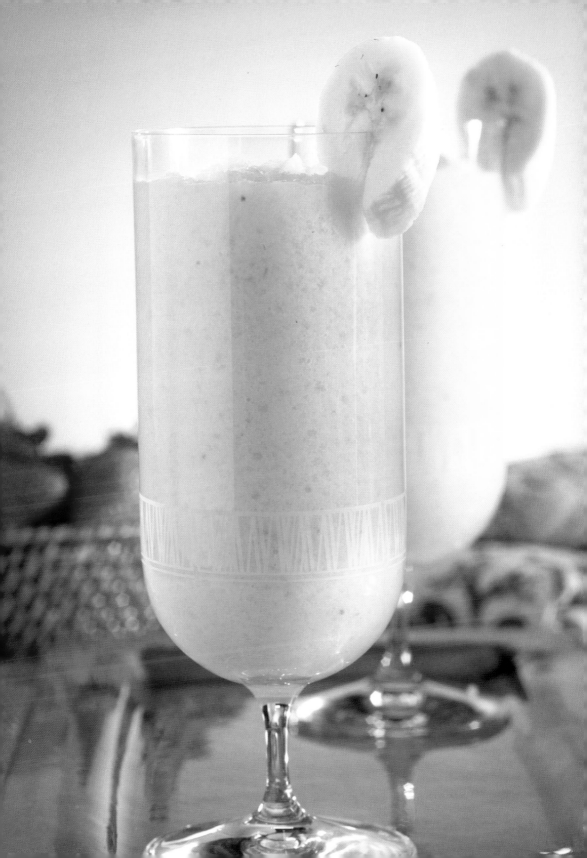

KIWI PINEAPPLE CREAM
MAKES 2 SERVINGS

¾ cup unsweetened coconut milk

1½ cups fresh pineapple chunks

2 kiwis, peeled and quartered

Grated peel and juice of 1 lime

Combine coconut milk, pineapple, kiwis, lime peel and lime juice in blender; blend until smooth.

KIWI CHAI SMOOTHIE

Add ¼ teaspoon vanilla, ⅛ teaspoon ground cardamom, ⅛ teaspoon ground cinnamon, ⅛ teaspoon ground ginger and a pinch of ground cloves to the mixture before blending.

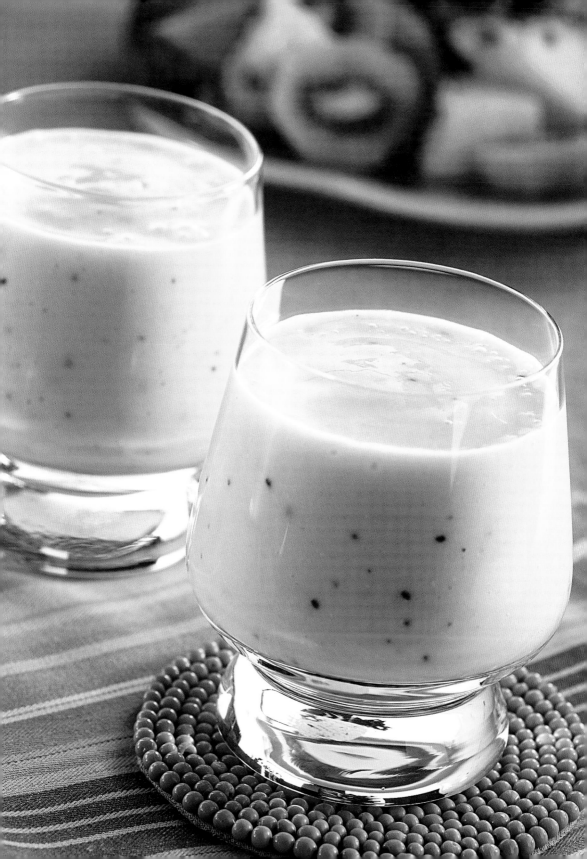

TROPICAL BREEZE SMOOTHIE
MAKES 2 SERVINGS

½ cup unsweetened coconut milk

1 cup frozen pineapple chunks

1 cup frozen mango chunks

1 tablespoon honey

Combine coconut milk, pineapple, mango and honey in blender; blend until smooth.

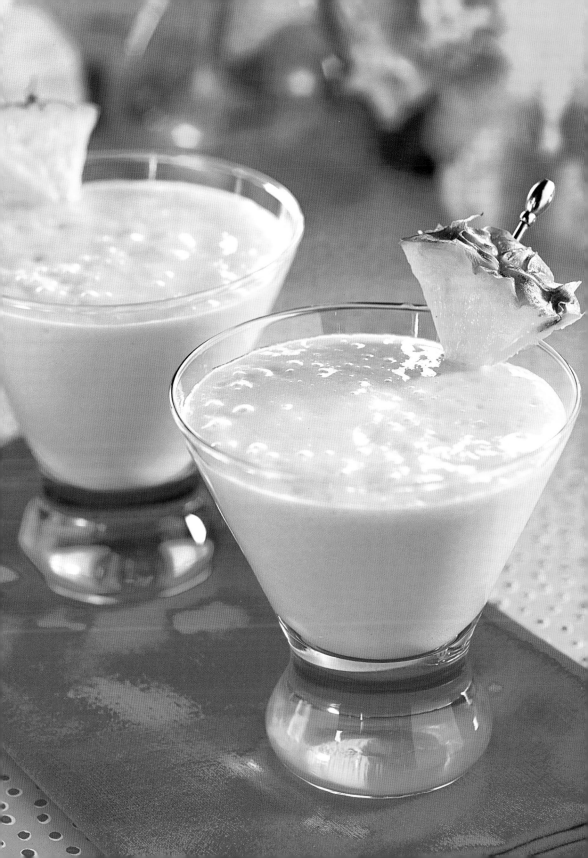

REFRESHING GREEN SMOOTHIE >
MAKES 1 SERVING

¾ cup unsweetened coconut milk

1 cup baby spinach

¾ cup frozen pineapple chunks

½ teaspoon grated lemon peel

Combine coconut milk, spinach, pineapple and lemon peel in blender; blend until smooth.

TROPICAL MANGO TANGO
MAKES 3 SERVINGS

1¼ cups coconut water

1½ cups frozen mango chunks

½ cup frozen pineapple chunks

½ banana

1 teaspoon grated fresh ginger

Combine coconut water, mango, pineapple, banana and ginger in blender; blend until smooth.

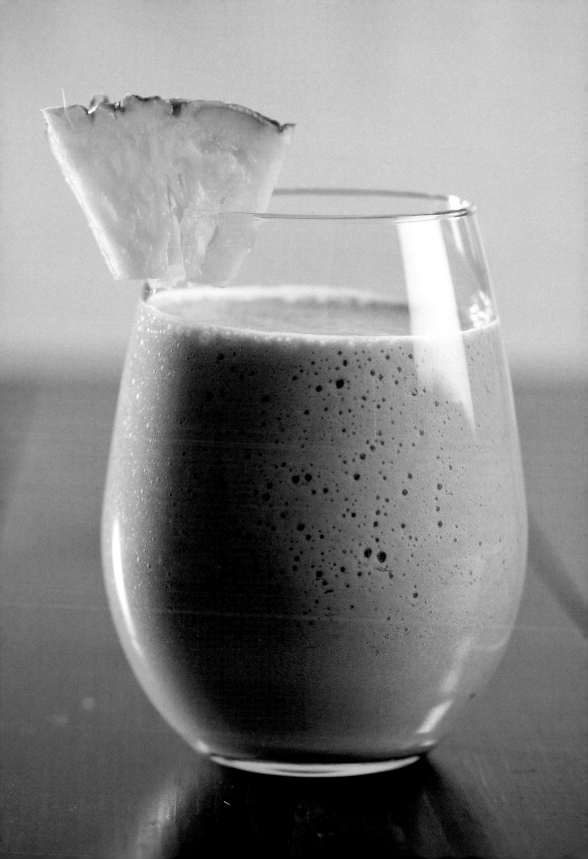

CUBAN BATIDO
MAKES 3 SERVINGS

- ¾ cup unsweetened coconut milk
- ½ cup orange juice
- 1½ cups fresh pineapple chunks
- 1 cup ice cubes
- 1 tablespoon lime juice

Combine coconut milk, orange juice, pineapple, ice and lime juice in blender; blend until smooth.

NOTE

A batido is a popular Latin American drink made with water, milk, fruit and ice. It is similar in texture to a smoothie and literally means "beaten" in Portuguese.

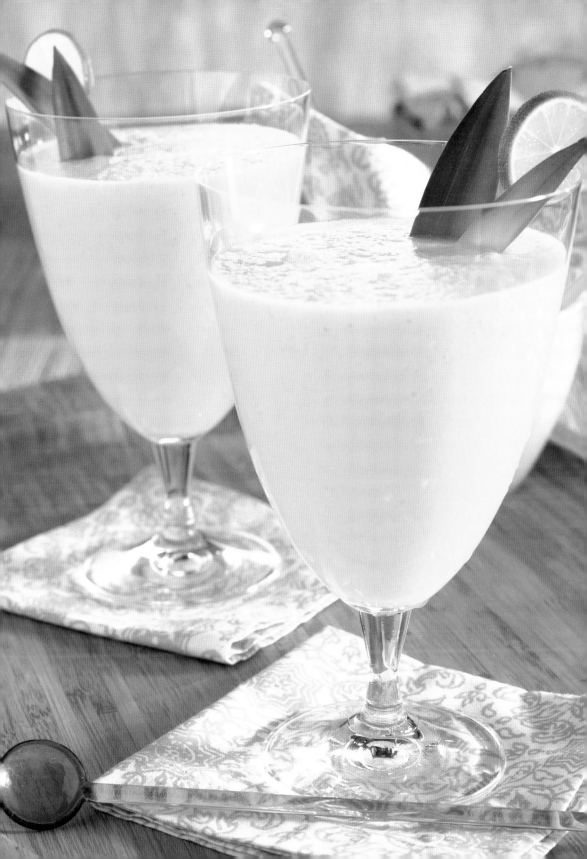

KIWI MANGO MAGIC
MAKES 2 SERVINGS

1 cup water

2 kiwis, peeled and quartered

¾ cup frozen pineapple chunks

¾ cup frozen mango chunks

⅓ cup fresh mint

Combine water, kiwis, pineapple, mango and mint in blender; blend until smooth.

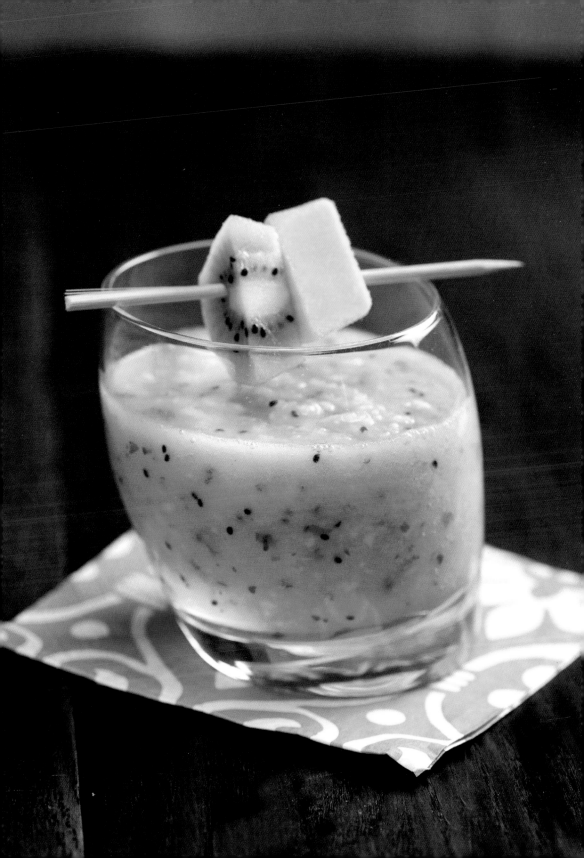

SUPERFOOD SMOOTHIES

POMEGRANATE FRUIT FLING
MAKES 2 SERVINGS

¼ cup water

1 navel orange, peeled and seeded

1 small pear, seeded and cut into chunks

½ cup pomegranate seeds

¼ cup ice cubes

Combine water, orange, pear, pomegranate seeds and ice in blender; blend until smooth.

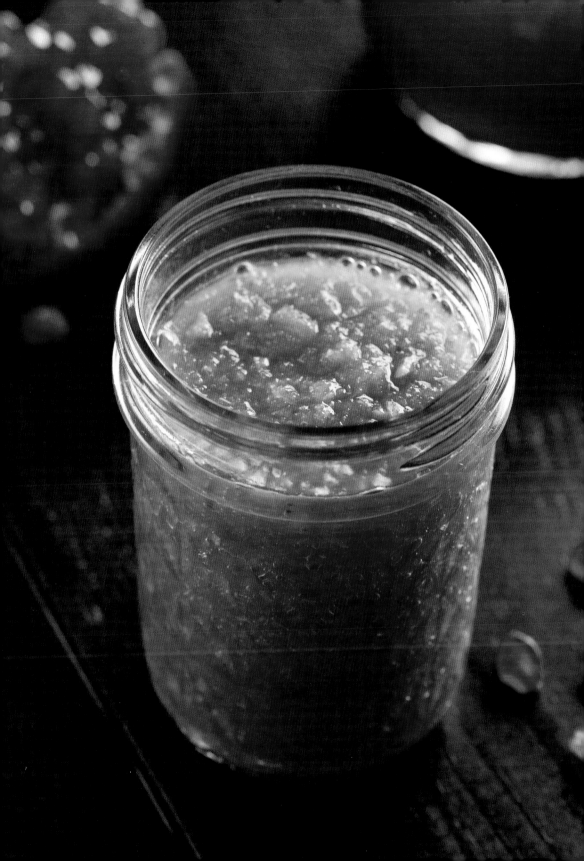

SPICED PUMPKIN BANANA SMOOTHIE
MAKES 1 SERVING

½ cup unsweetened almond milk

½ frozen banana

½ cup ice cubes

½ cup canned pumpkin

1 tablespoon honey

1 teaspoon ground flaxseed

¼ teaspoon ground cinnamon

⅛ teaspoon ground ginger

   Dash ground nutmeg

Combine almond milk, banana, ice, pumpkin, honey, flaxseed, cinnamon, ginger and nutmeg in blender; blend until smooth.

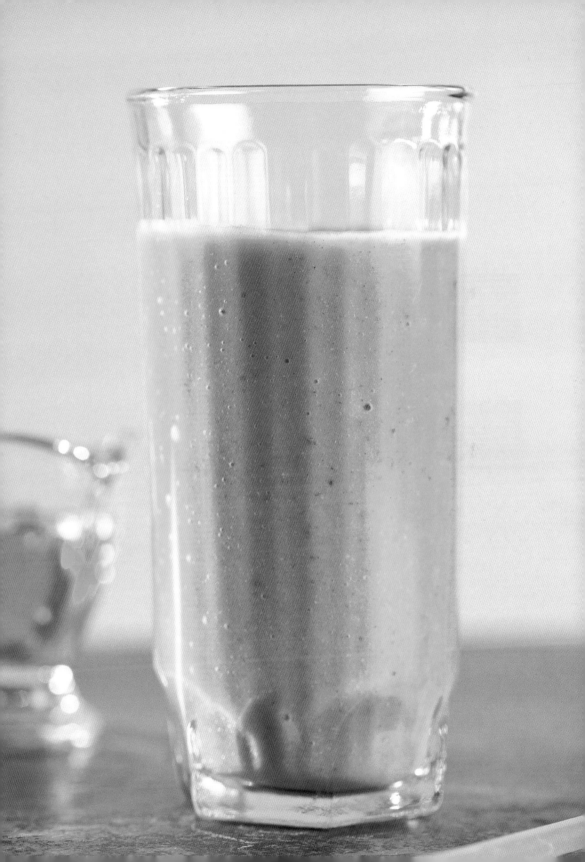

AUTUMN CELEBRATION SMOOTHIE
MAKES 2 SERVINGS

2 plums, pitted and cut into chunks

1 pear, seeded and cut into chunks

½ cup fresh or thawed frozen cranberries

¼ cup ice cubes

⅛ teaspoon ground ginger

⅛ teaspoon ground cinnamon

Combine plums, pear, cranberries, ice, ginger and cinnamon in blender; blend until smooth. Serve immediately.

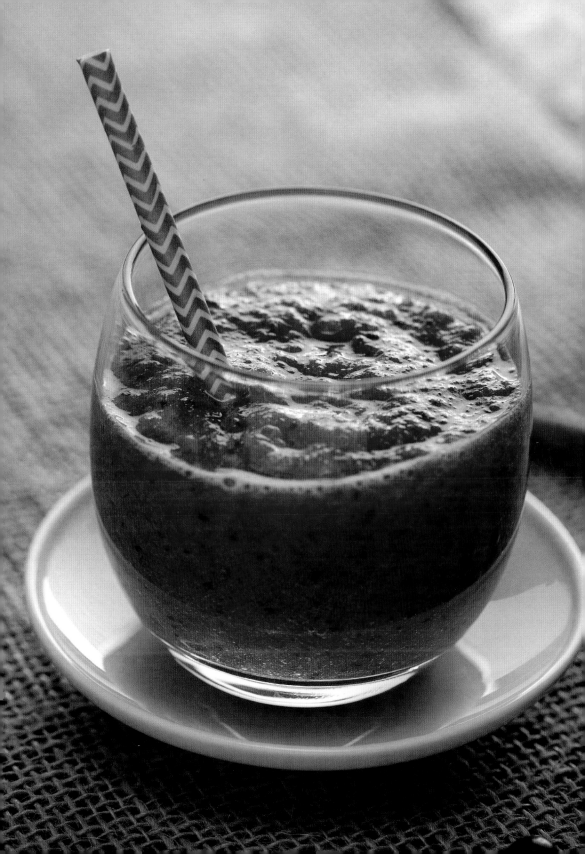

BLACKBERRY LIME SMOOTHIE
MAKES 1 SERVING

½ cup unsweetened coconut milk

1 cup fresh blackberries

2 ice cubes

1 tablespoon lime juice

2 teaspoons honey

½ teaspoon grated lime peel

Combine coconut milk, blackberries, ice, lime juice, honey and lime peel in blender; blend until smooth.

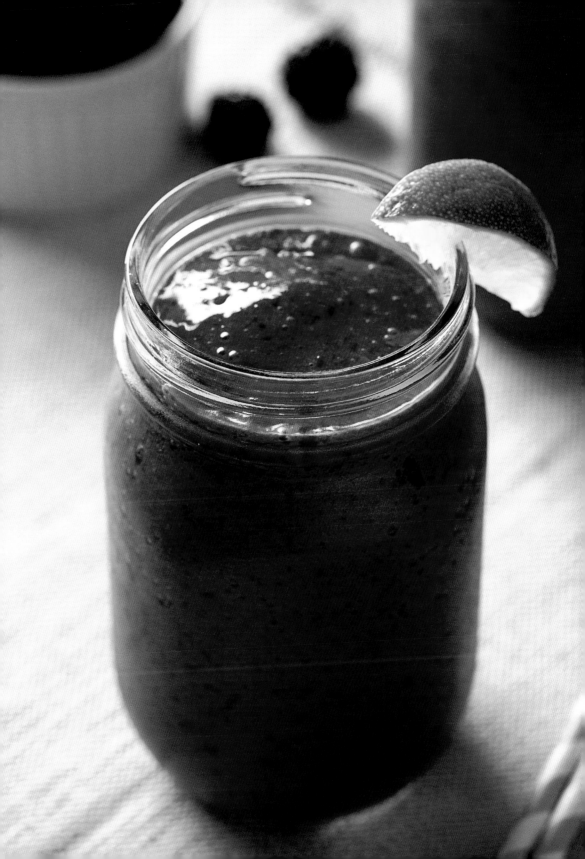

SUPER SMOOTHIE >

MAKES 1 SERVING

- ½ cup apple juice
- 1 cup packed stemmed kale
- 1 cup baby spinach
- 1 banana
- 1 cup ice cubes

Combine apple juice, kale, spinach, banana and ice in blender; blend until smooth.

AVOCADO BANANA SMOOTHIE

MAKES 1 SERVING

- ½ cup water
- 1 frozen banana
- 1 avocado, pitted and peeled
- ⅓ cup baby spinach
- 2 teaspoons honey
- ¼ teaspoon grated lemon peel

Combine ½ cup water, banana, avocado, spinach, honey and lemon peel in blender; blend until smooth. Add additional water, 1 tablespoon at at time, until desired consistency is reached.

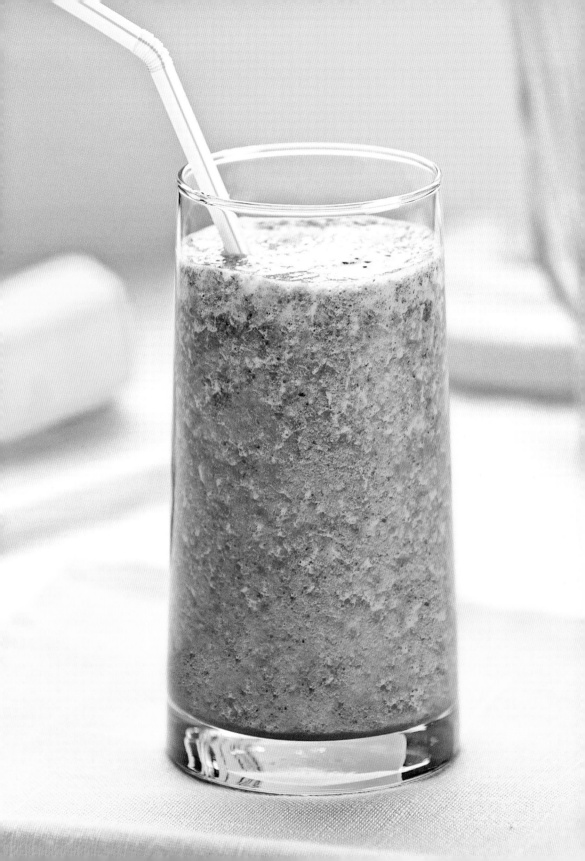

BEET AND BERRY BLAST
MAKES 2 SERVINGS

- ¾ cup orange juice
- ¾ cup canned sliced beets
- ¾ cup frozen mixed berries
- ¾ cup ice cubes
- 1½ tablespoons lemon juice
- 1½ tablespoons honey

Combine orange juice, beets, berries, ice, lemon juice and honey in blender; blend until smooth.

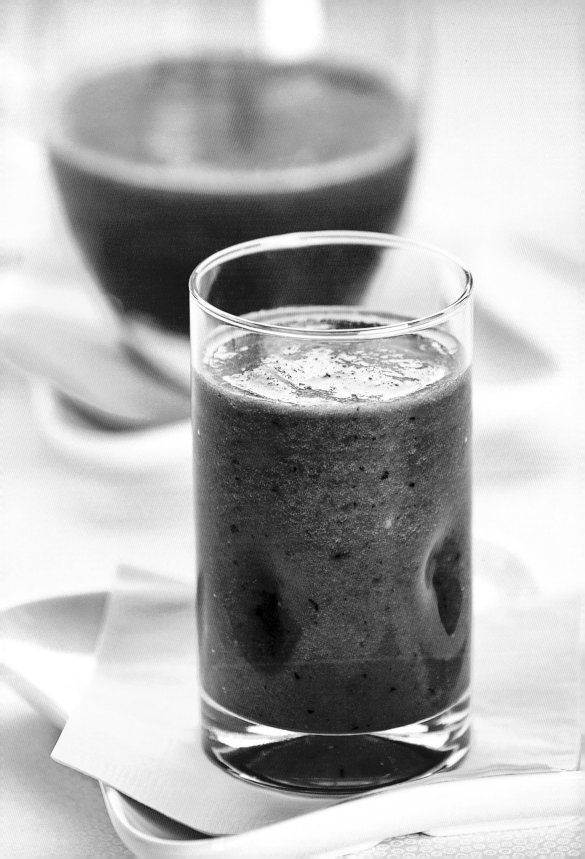

SUPER BLUE SMOOTHIE
MAKES 2 SERVINGS

½ **cup pomegranate juice**

¼ **cup water**

¾ **cup frozen blueberries**

¾ **cup frozen blackberries**

½ **avocado, pitted and peeled**

2 **teaspoons honey**

Combine pomegranate juice, water, blueberries, blackberries, avocado and honey in blender; blend until smooth.

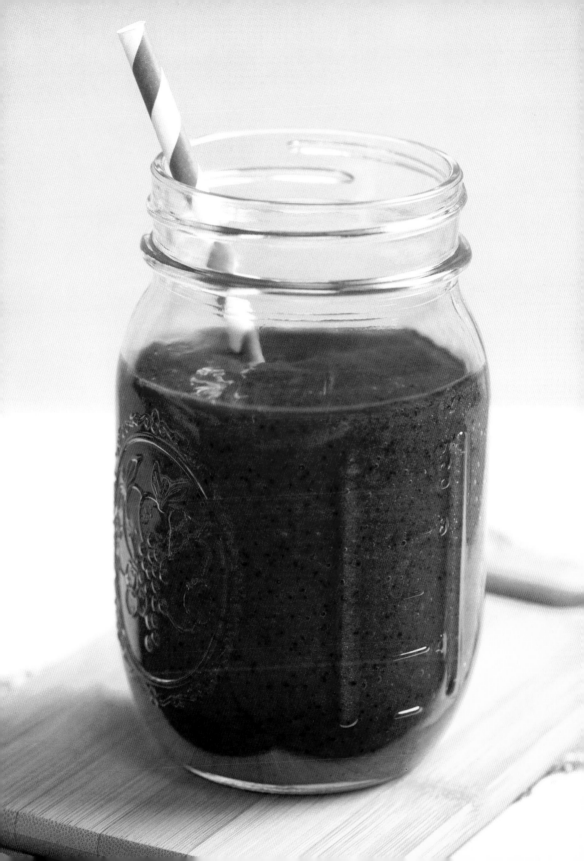

SALAD BAR SMOOTHIE

MAKES 1 SERVING

1½ cups ice cubes

½ banana

½ cup fresh raspberries

½ cup sliced fresh strawberries

½ cup fresh blueberries

½ cup packed spinach

Combine ice, banana, raspberries, strawberries, blueberries and spinach in blender; blend until smooth.

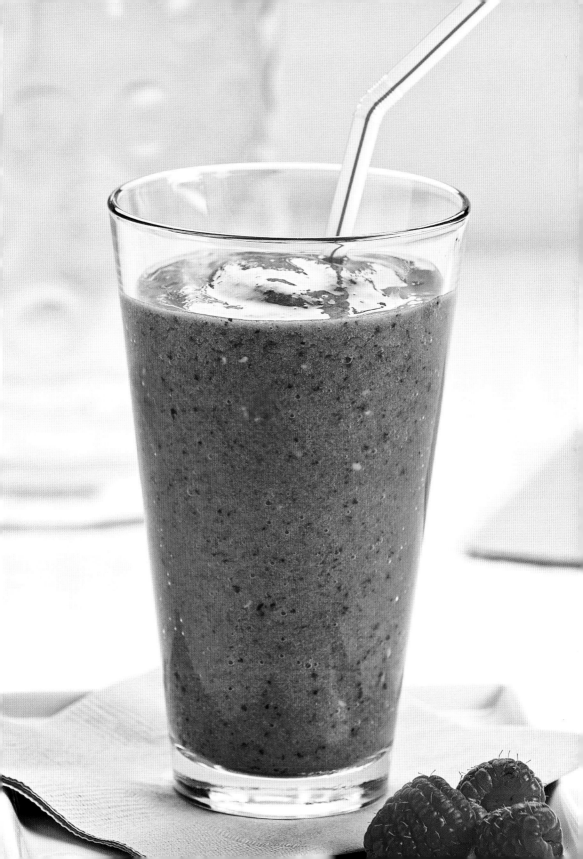

CINNAMON SQUASH PEAR SMOOTHIE >

MAKES 1 SERVING

1 pear, seeded and cut into chunks

¾ cup frozen cooked winter squash

1 teaspoon honey

¼ teaspoon ground cinnamon

Combine pear, squash, honey and cinnamon in blender; blend until smooth.

BLUE KALE SMOOTHIE

MAKES 2 SERVINGS

¼ cup unsweetened almond milk

1 cup packed stemmed kale

1 frozen banana

½ cup fresh blueberries

¼ cup ice cubes

Combine almond milk, kale, banana, blueberries and ice in blender; blend until smooth.

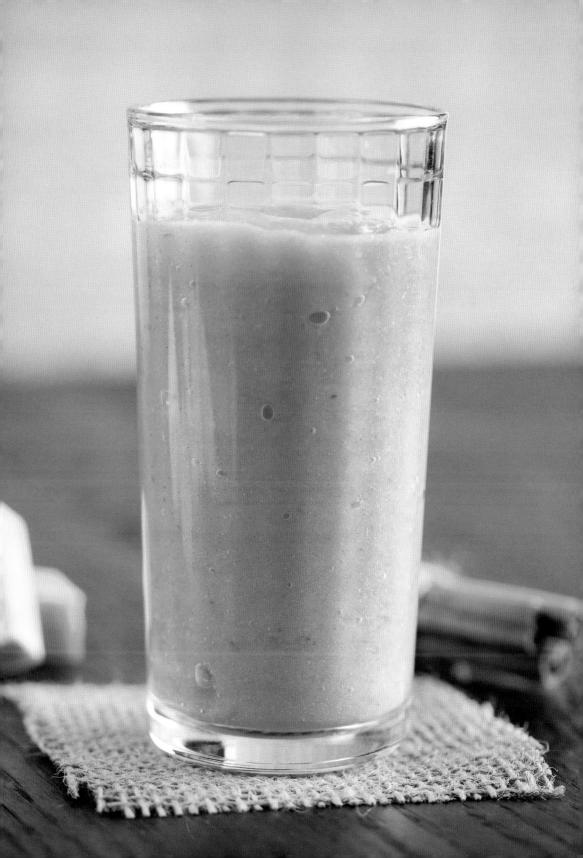

CHERRY BERRY POMEGRANATE SMOOTHIE
MAKES 2 SERVINGS

¾ cup water

1 cup frozen dark sweet cherries

½ cup frozen strawberries

½ cup pomegranate seeds

1 tablespoon chia seeds

1 teaspoon lemon juice

Combine water, cherries, strawberries, pomegranate seeds, chia seeds and lemon juice in blender; blend until smooth.

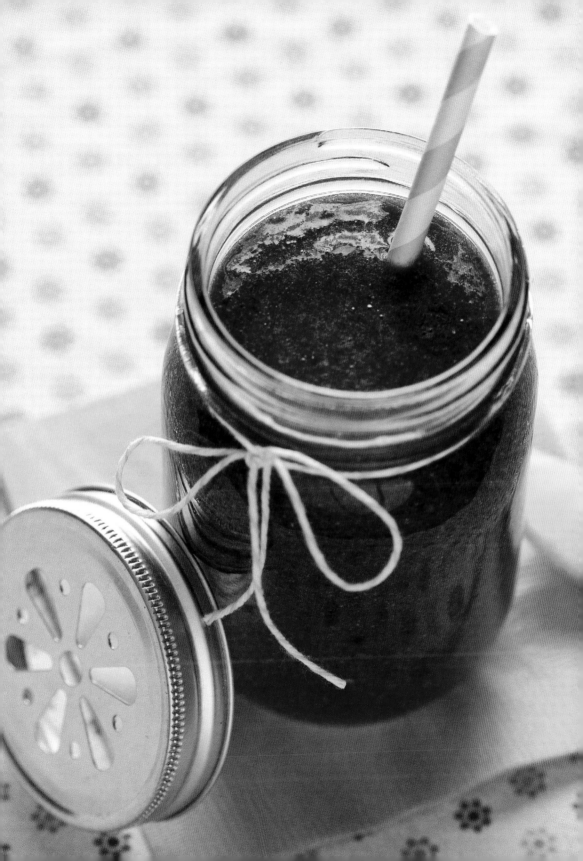

GREEN GOODNESS
MAKES 3 SERVINGS

2 pears, seeded and cut into chunks

2 cups baby kale

1 avocado, pitted and peeled

1 cup ice cubes

½ cup fresh mint

Combine pears, kale, avocado, ice and mint in blender; blend until smooth.

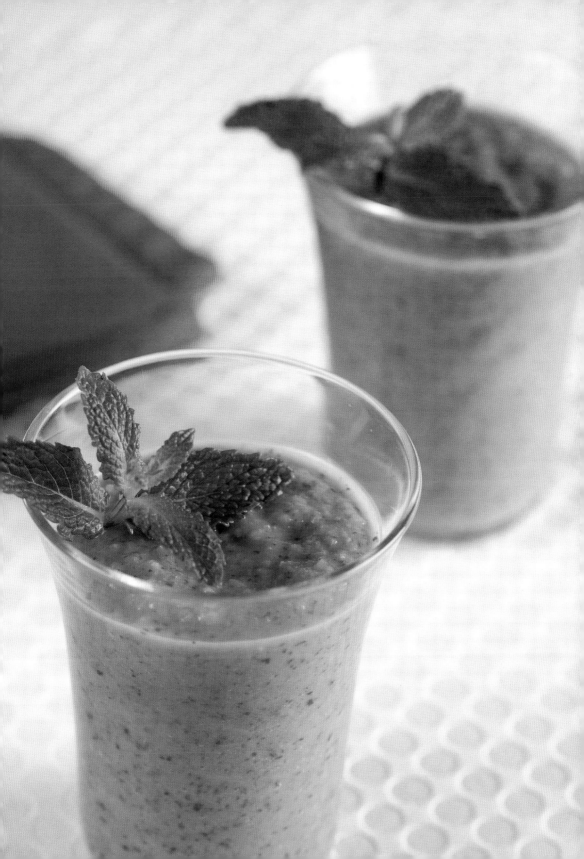

CHOCOLATE BLUEBERRY SHAKE
MAKES 1 SERVING

¼ **cup unsweetened almond milk**

½ **cup fresh blueberries**

¼ **cup ice cubes**

2 **teaspoons honey**

½ **teaspoon unsweetened cocoa powder**

Combine almond milk, blueberries, ice, honey and cocoa in blender; blend until smooth.

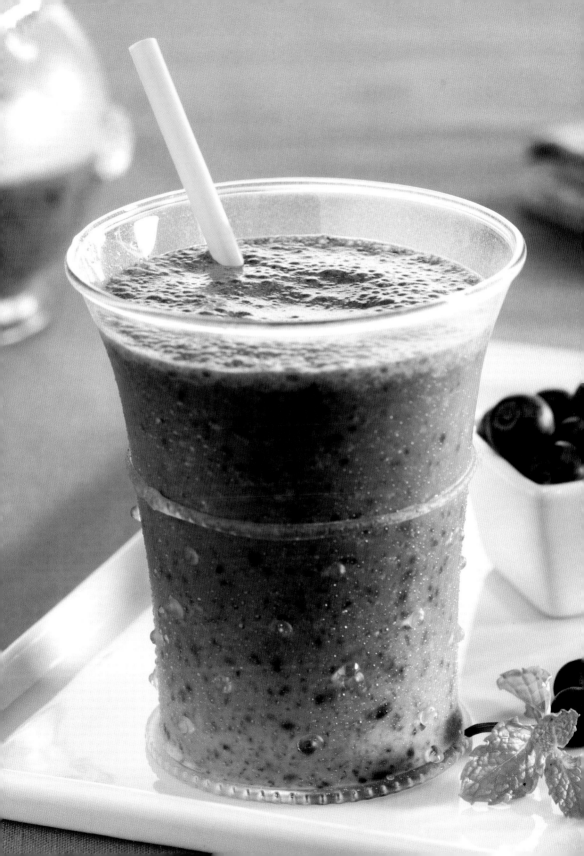

IMMUNITY BOOSTERS

CRAN-ORANGE RASPBERRY SMOOTHIE
MAKES 2 SERVINGS

¼ cup water

2 navel oranges, peeled and seeded

½ cup fresh or thawed frozen cranberries

½ cup frozen raspberries

2 teaspoons honey

Combine water, oranges, cranberries, raspberries and honey in blender; blend until smooth.

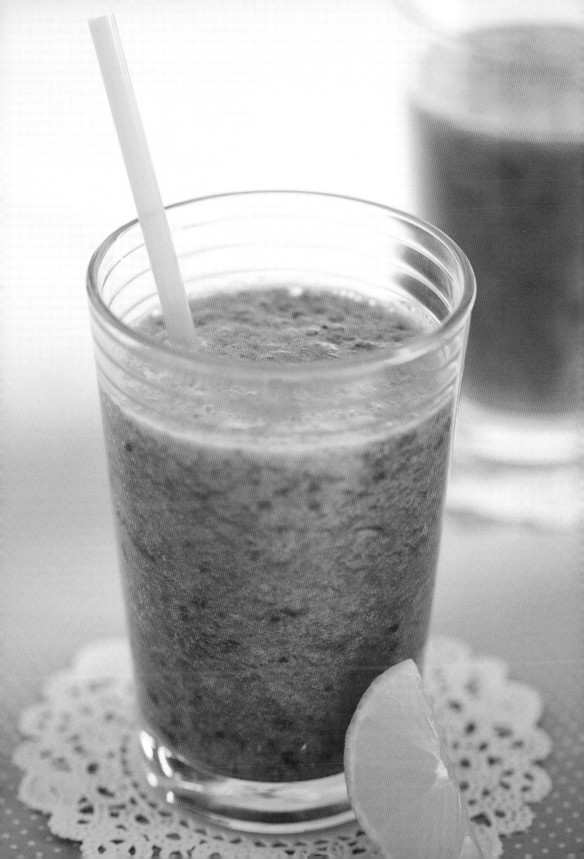

STRAWBERRY BASIL COOLER
MAKES 2 SERVINGS

- 1 cup water
- 1¼ cups frozen strawberries
- ½ cup ice cubes
- ¼ cup fresh basil leaves
- 2 teaspoons lemon juice
- 2 teaspoons honey

Combine water, strawberries, ice, basil, lemon juice and honey in blender; blend until smooth.

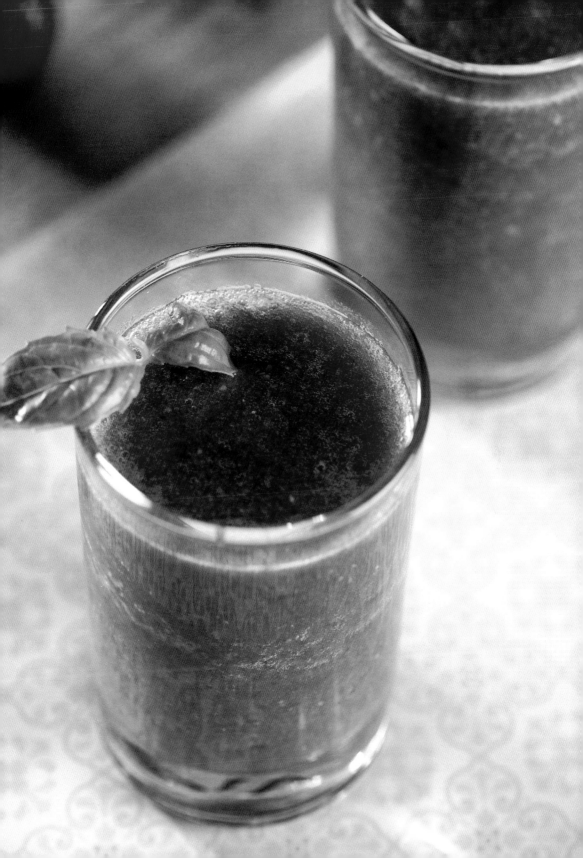

BLUEBERRY PEACH BLISS

MAKES 2 SERVINGS

1¼ cups water

1 cup frozen blueberries

1 cup frozen sliced peaches

1 tablespoon lemon juice

2 teaspoons honey

½ teaspoon grated fresh ginger

Combine water, blueberries, peaches, lemon juice, honey and ginger in blender; blend until smooth.

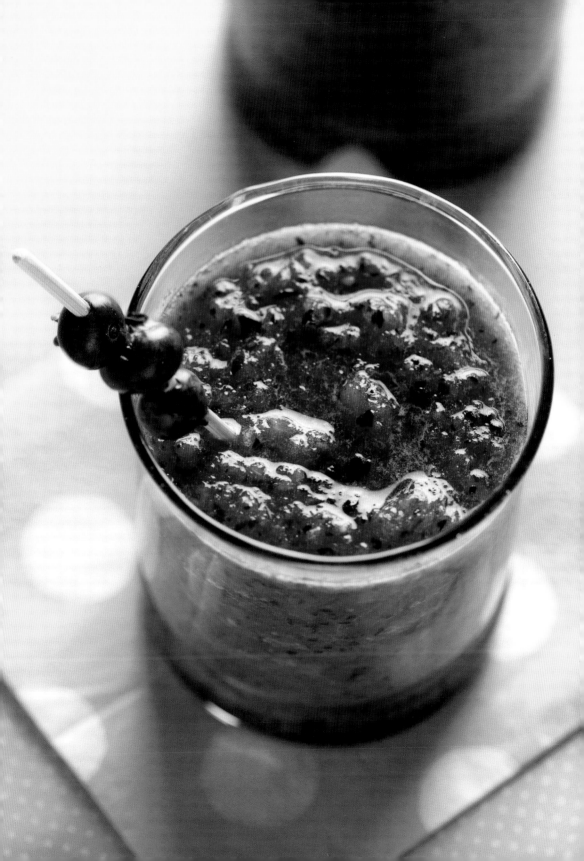

BERRY CRANBERRY BLAST

MAKES 2 SERVINGS

1 cup water

1 cup frozen mixed berries

½ cup fresh or thawed frozen cranberries

½ avocado, pitted and peeled

1 tablespoon honey

½ teaspoon grated fresh ginger

Combine water, mixed berries, cranberries, avocado, honey and ginger in blender; blend until smooth.

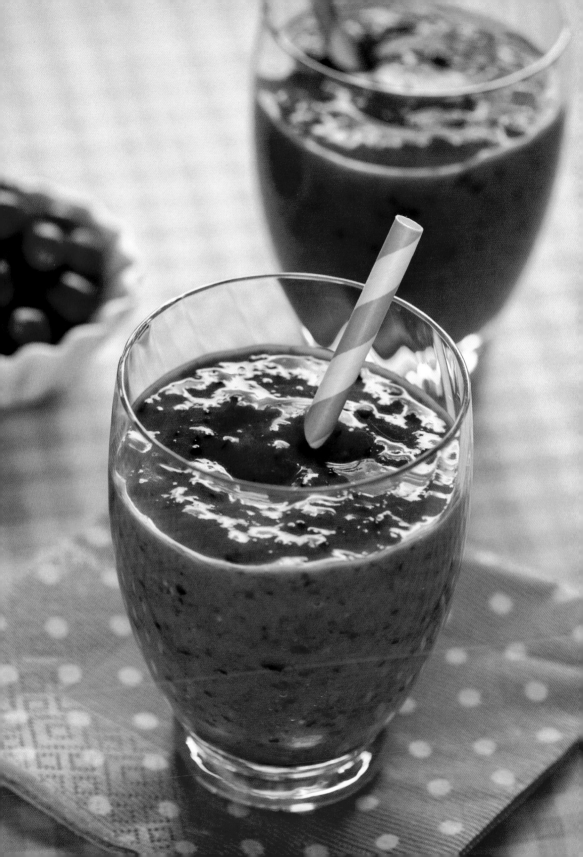

BLUEBERRY APPLE BOOSTER
MAKES 2 SERVINGS

½ cup apple juice

1½ cups frozen blueberries

1 Granny Smith apple, seeded and cut into chunks

⅛ teaspoon ground allspice

Combine apple juice, blueberries, apple and allspice in blender; blend until smooth.

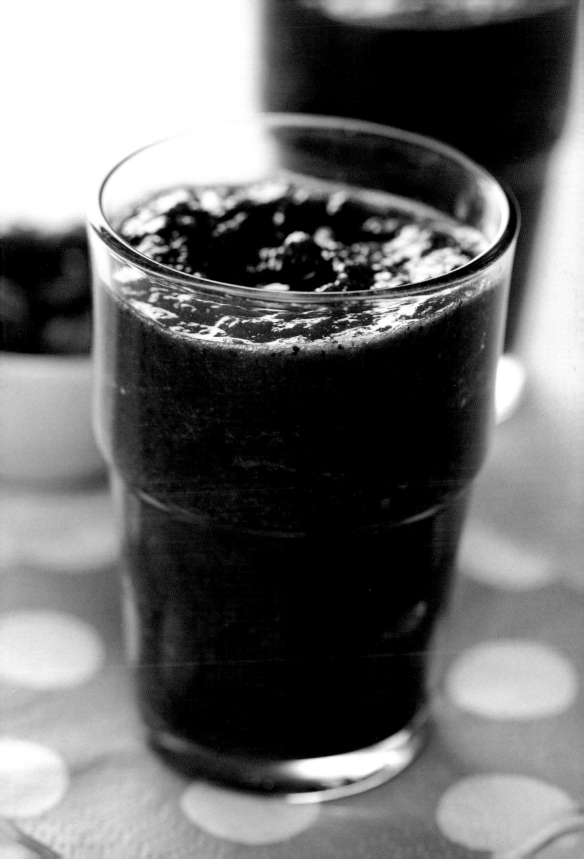

MIXED BERRY BLEND >
MAKES 2 SERVINGS

1 cup apple juice

1½ cups sliced fresh strawberries

1 cup fresh blueberries

½ cup fresh raspberries

½ cup ice cubes

Combine apple juice, strawberries, blueberries, raspberries and ice in blender; blend until smooth.

FROZEN WATERMELON WHIP
MAKES 2 SERVINGS

1 cup brewed lemon herbal tea, at room temperature

1¾ cups ice cubes

1½ cups seedless watermelon chunks

Combine tea, ice and watermelon in blender; blend until smooth. Serve immediately.

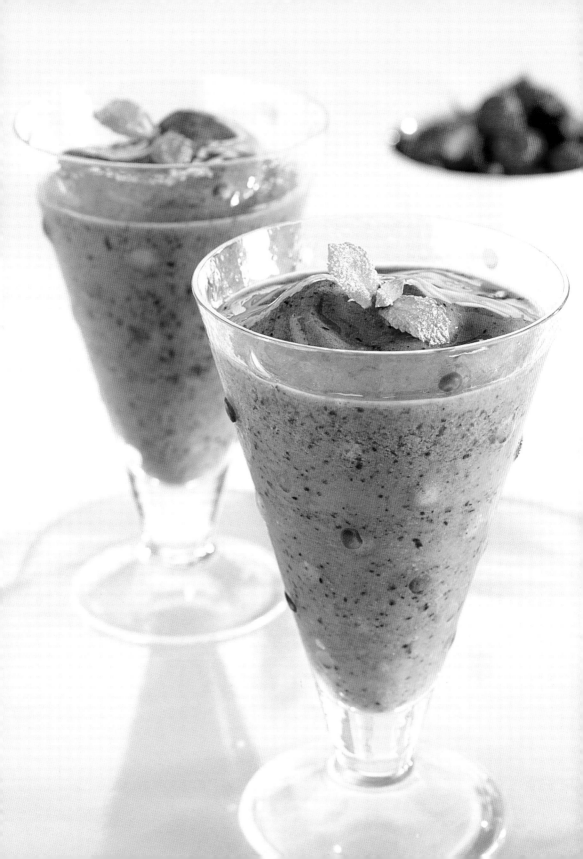

SUPER C SMOOTHIE
MAKES 3 SERVINGS

⅔ cup water

2 navel oranges, peeled and seeded

2 cups baby kale

2 cups frozen blackberries

1 avocado, pitted and peeled

2 tablespoons honey

Combine water, oranges, kale, blackberries, avocado and honey in blender; blend until smooth.

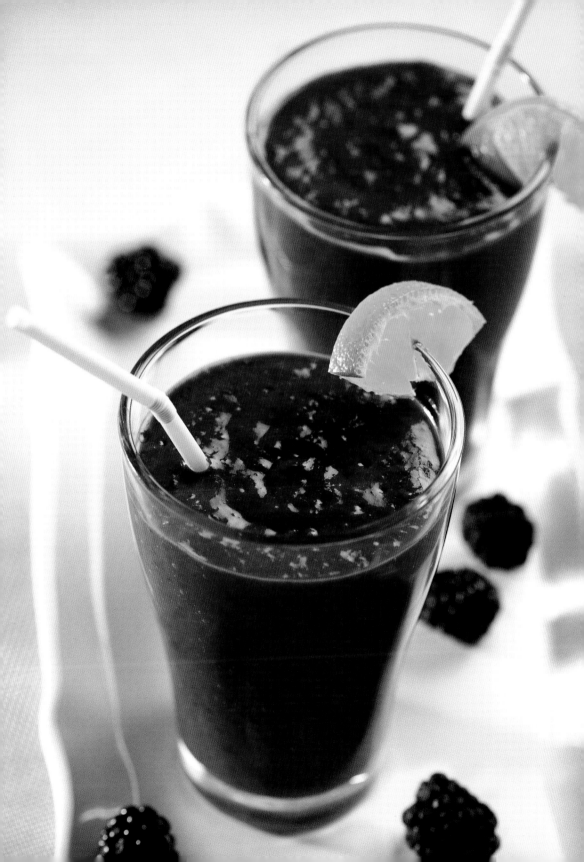

SPA SMOOTHIE

MAKES 3 SERVINGS

1 cup peeled cucumber chunks

1 cup cantaloupe chunks

1 cup sliced fresh strawberries

1 cup ice cubes

Grated peel and juice of 2 lemons

2 tablespoons honey

Combine cucumber, cantaloupe, strawberries, ice, lemon peel, lemon juice and honey in blender; blend until smooth.

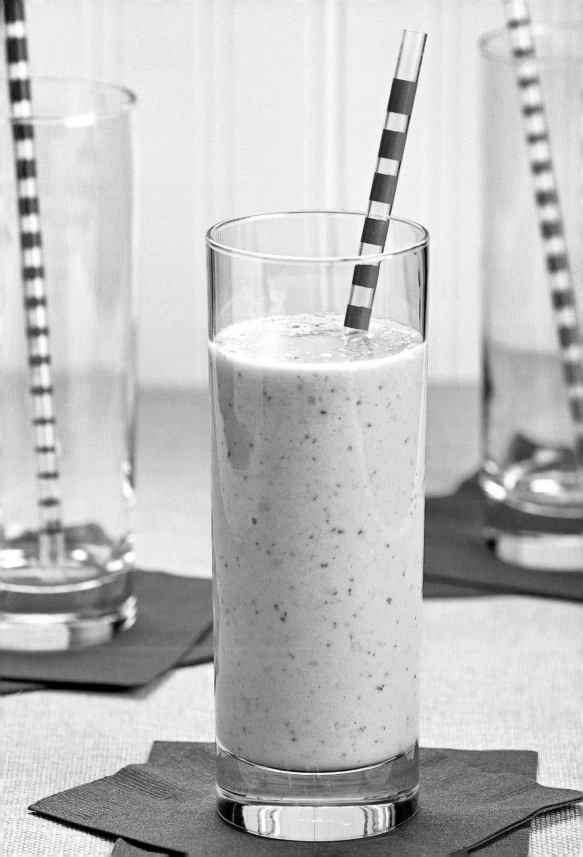

GRAPE STRAWBERRY SUNSET

MAKES 2 SERVINGS

½ cup water

1 sweet red apple, seeded and cut into chunks

1 cup frozen red seedless grapes

1 cup frozen strawberries

1 teaspoon lemon juice

Combine water, apple, grapes, strawberries and lemon juice in blender; blend until smooth.

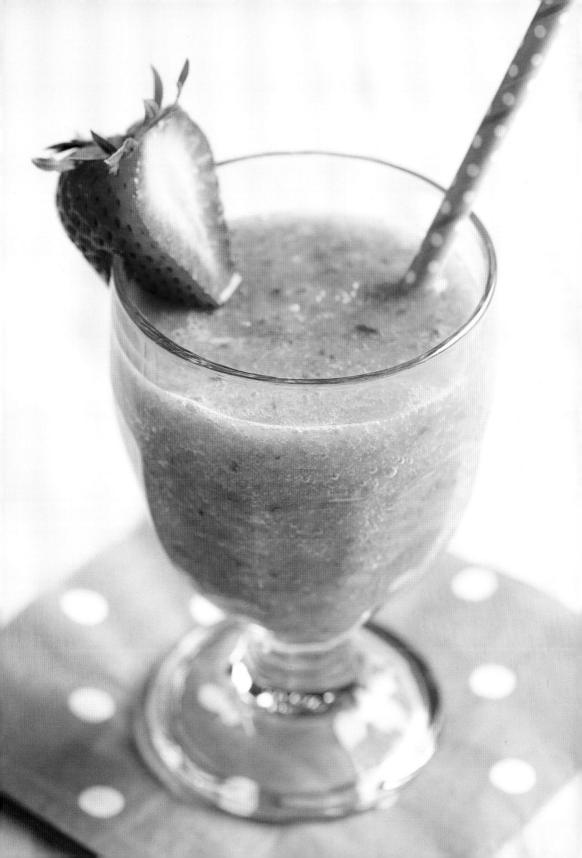

CHERRY ALMOND SMOOTHIE
MAKES 2 SERVINGS

½ cup unsweetened almond milk

1½ cups frozen dark sweet cherries

½ banana

2 teaspoons almond butter

⅛ teaspoon ground cinnamon

Combine almond milk, cherries, banana, almond butter and cinnamon in blender; blend until smooth.

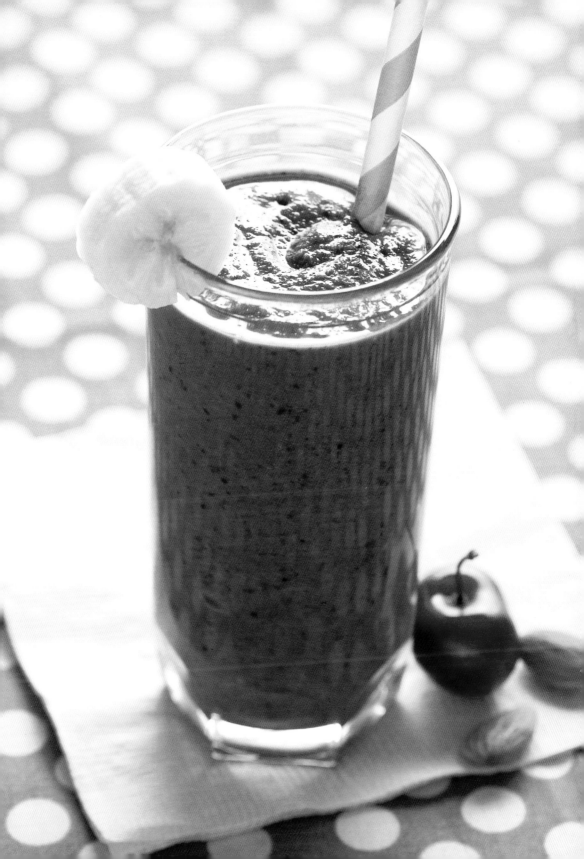

ORANGE APRICOT SUNSHINE
MAKES 2 SERVINGS

½ **cup dried apricots**

¾ **cup water**

1 **navel orange, peeled and seeded**

½ **cup frozen mango chunks**

½ **teaspoon grated fresh ginger**

1 Place apricots in small bowl; cover with hot water. Let stand 10 minutes; drain.

2 Combine water, orange, mango, apricots and ginger in blender; blend until smooth.

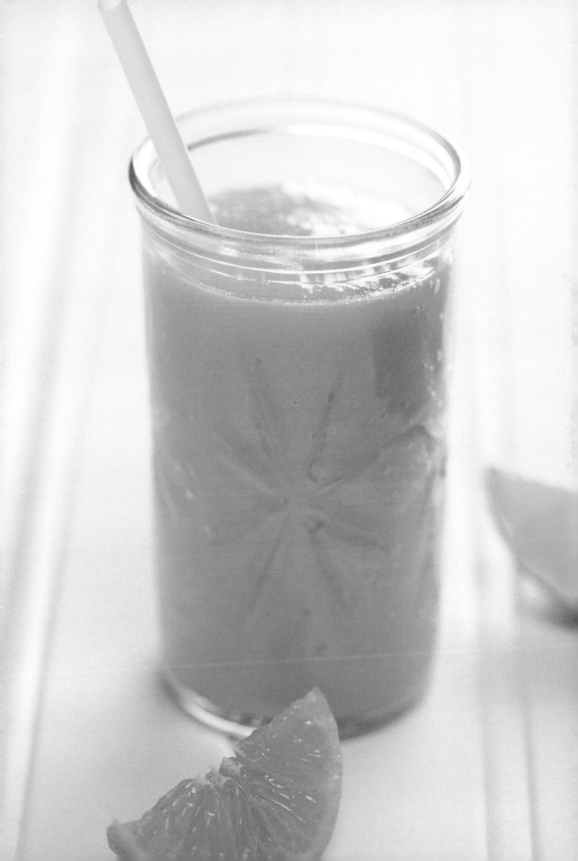

BERRY TANGERINE DREAM
MAKES 3 SERVINGS

- ½ cup water
- 2 tangerines, peeled and seeded
- 2 cups frozen mixed berries
- 1 cup fresh pineapple chunks
- 2 teaspoons honey

Combine water, tangerines, mixed berries, pineapple and honey in blender; blend until smooth.

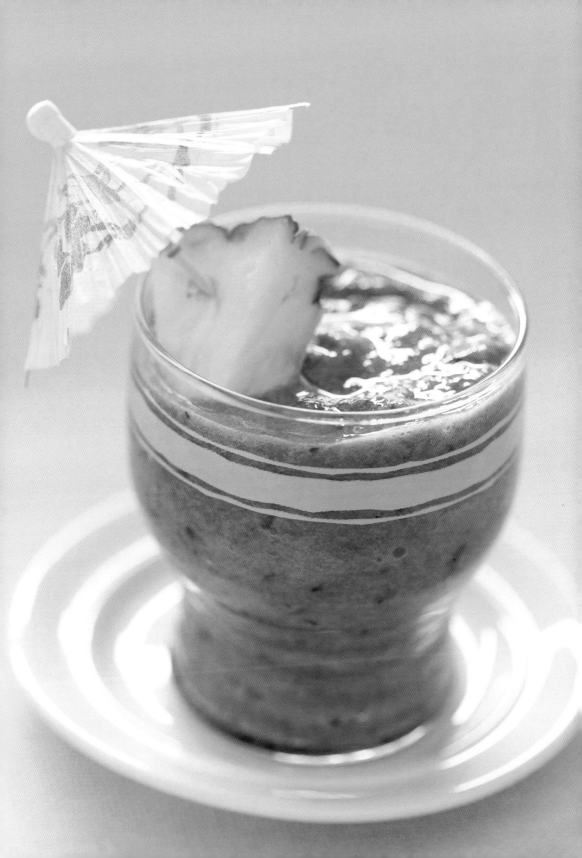

ENERGIZING SMOOTHIES

BERRY MOJITO SMOOTHIE
MAKES 2 SERVINGS

1¼ cups water

1 cup frozen strawberries

½ cup frozen raspberries

1 tablespoon lime juice

1 tablespoon honey

½ cup fresh mint

Combine water, strawberries, raspberries, lime juice, honey and mint in blender; blend until smooth.

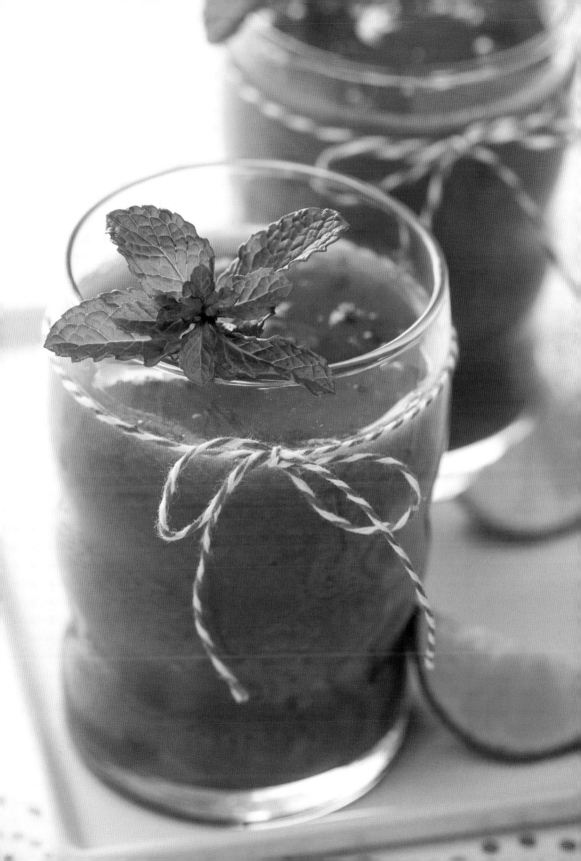

BLUEBERRY CHERRY BLEND

MAKES 2 SERVINGS

¾ cup water

¾ cup frozen blueberries

¾ cup frozen dark sweet cherries

½ avocado, pitted and peeled

1 tablespoon lemon juice

1 teaspoon ground flaxseed

Combine water, blueberries, cherries, avocado, lemon juice and flaxseed in blender; blend until smooth.

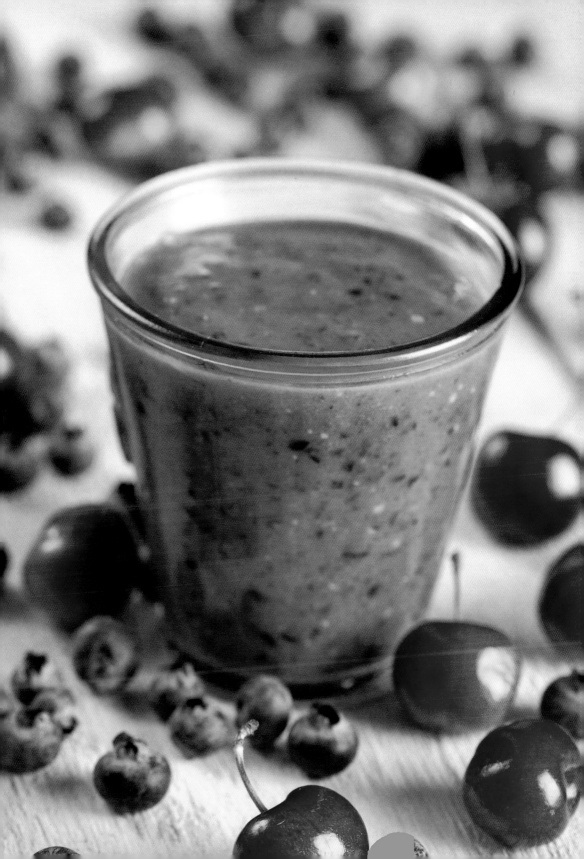

LEMON STRAWBERRY SMOOTHIE
MAKES 1 SERVING

¾ cup unsweetened almond milk

1 cup sliced fresh strawberries

¼ cup ice cubes

1 tablespoon honey

1 tablespoon lemon juice

1 teaspoon grated lemon peel

Combine almond milk, strawberries, ice, honey, lemon juice and lemon peel in blender; blend until smooth.

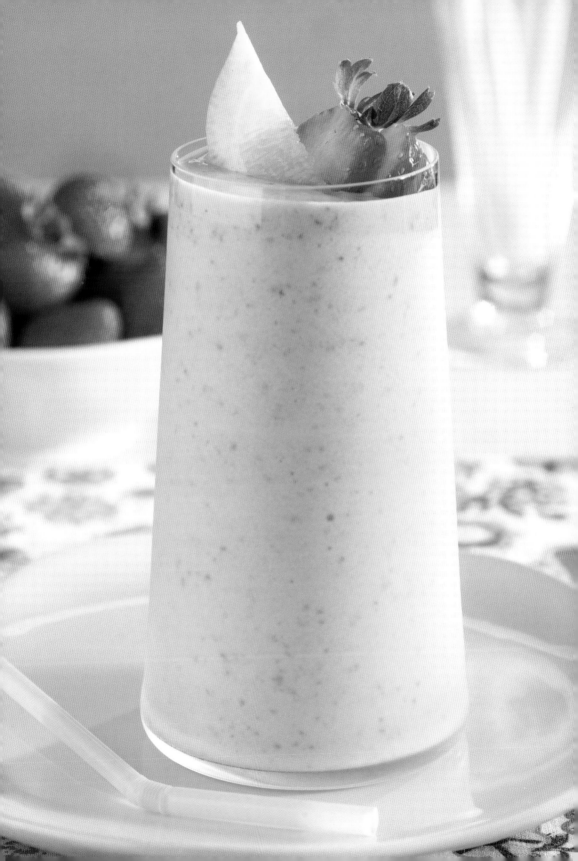

KIWI GREEN DREAM

MAKES 2 SERVINGS

¾ **cup water**

2 **kiwis, peeled and quartered**

½ **cup frozen pineapple chunks**

½ **avocado, pitted and peeled**

1 **tablespoon chia seeds**

Combine water, kiwis, pineapple, avocado and chia seeds in blender; blend until smooth.

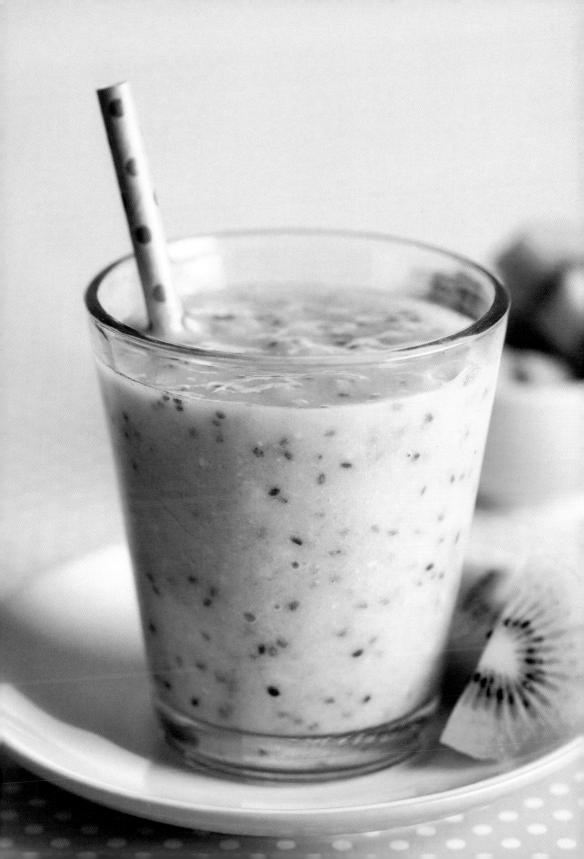

PURPLE PICK-ME-UP >
MAKES 2 SERVINGS

¼ cup water

1 navel orange, peeled and seeded

1 cup frozen blueberries

4 medjool dates, pitted

Combine water, orange, blueberries and dates in blender; blend until smooth.

CHEERY CHERRY SMOOTHIE
MAKES 2 SERVINGS

1 cup unsweetened coconut milk

1 cup frozen sliced peaches

½ cup frozen dark sweet cherries

2 teaspoons lemon juice

Dash ground allspice

Combine coconut milk, peaches, cherries, lemon juice and allspice in blender; blend until smooth.

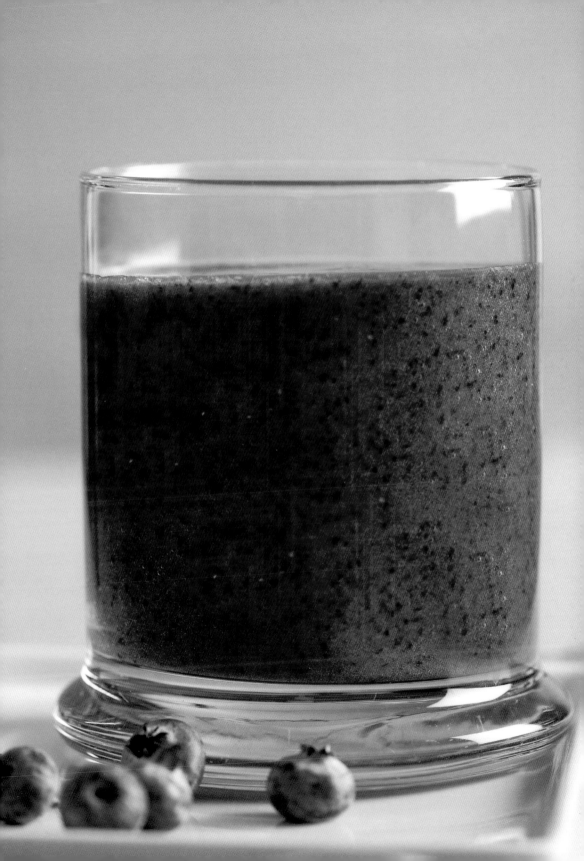

SWEET BEET TREAT

MAKES 2 SERVINGS

- ¼ cup water
- 2 carrots, cut into chunks
- 1 beet, peeled and cut into chunks
- 1 large sweet red apple, seeded and cut into chunks
- ¼ cup ice cubes
- 1 tablespoon lemon juice

Combine water, carrots, beet, apple, ice and lemon juice in blender; blend until smooth.

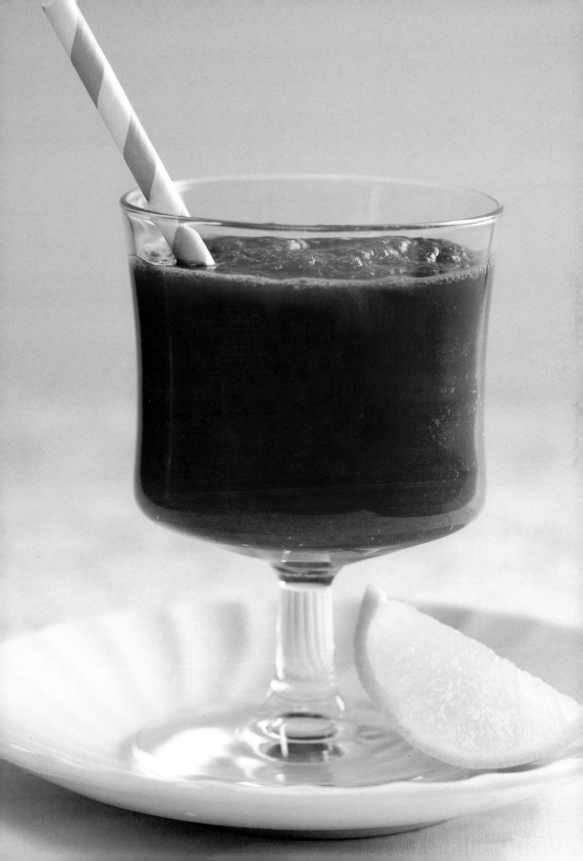

RASPBERRY LEMON BRAIN FREEZE

MAKES 2 SERVINGS

- ½ cup water
- ⅓ cup lemon juice (about 2 lemons)
- 1 cup ice cubes
- ¾ cup frozen raspberries
- 3 tablespoons honey

Combine water, lemon juice, ice, raspberries and honey in blender; blend until smooth.

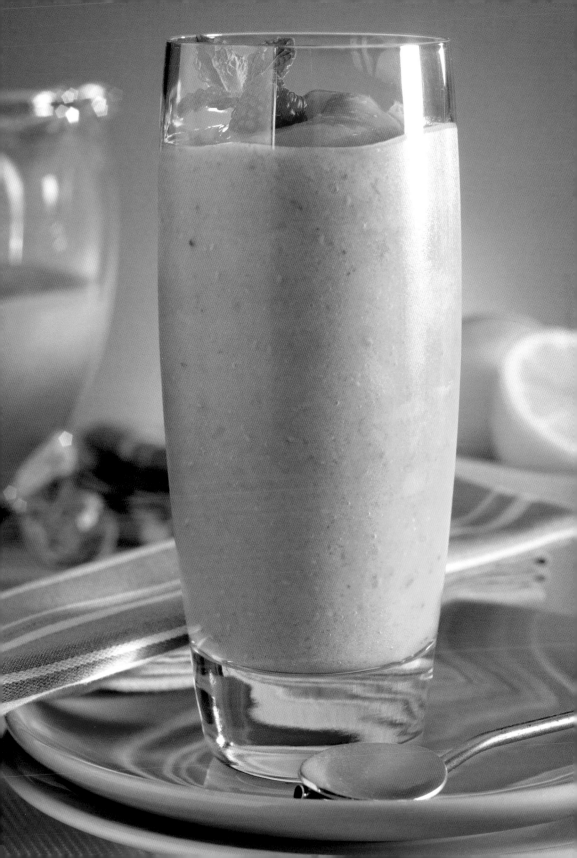

GREEN POWER SMOOTHIE
MAKES 3 SERVINGS

½ cup coconut water or water

2 cups packed spinach

1 cup fresh pineapple chunks

1 cup frozen mango chunks

½ frozen banana

Combine coconut water, spinach, pineapple, mango and banana in blender; blend until smooth.

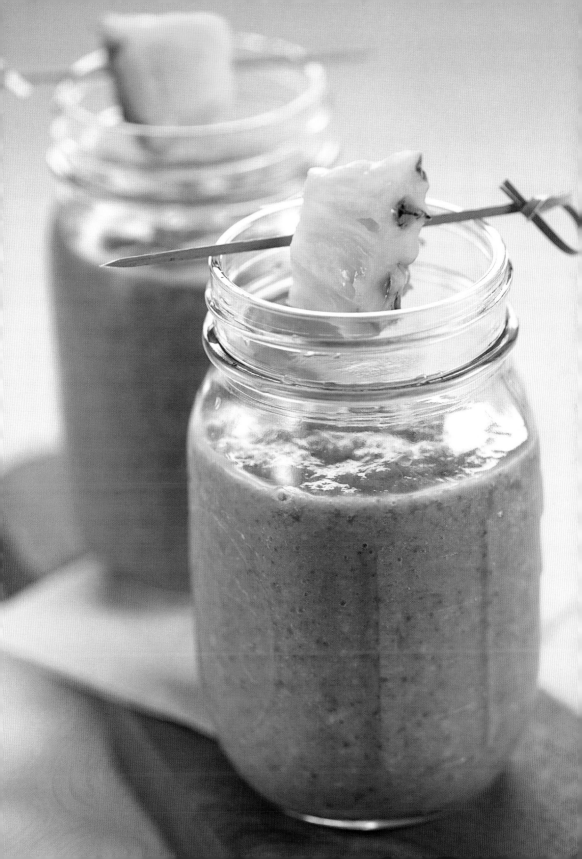

REFRESH SMOOTHIE >
MAKES 1 SERVING

½ cucumber, peeled, seeded and cut into chunks

1 cup frozen mixed berries

¼ cup ice cubes

1 tablespoon honey

Grated peel and juice of 1 lime

Combine cucumber, mixed berries, ice, honey, lime peel and lime juice in blender; blend until smooth.

ENERGY SMOOTHIE
MAKES 2 SERVINGS

½ cup unsweetened almond milk

1½ cups sliced fresh strawberries

1 frozen banana

2 tablespoons lemon juice

Combine almond milk, strawberries, banana and lemon juice in blender; blend until smooth.

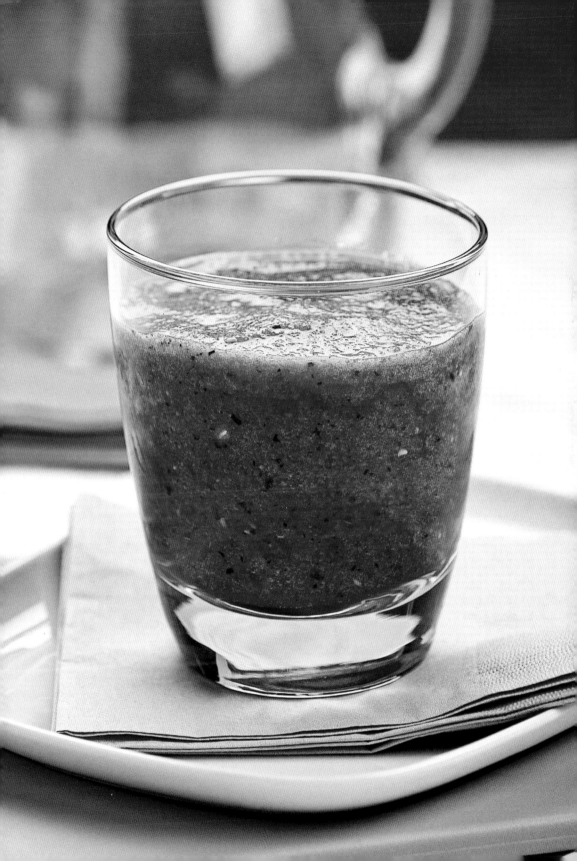

PUMPKIN POWER SMOOTHIE
MAKES 1 SERVING

⅓ cup water

1 sweet red apple, seeded and cut into chunks

½ frozen banana

½ cup ice cubes

½ cup canned pumpkin

1 tablespoon lemon juice

1 tablespoon ground flaxseed

1 teaspoon honey

Dash ground nutmeg

Combine water, apple, banana, ice, pumpkin, lemon juice, flaxseed, honey and nutmeg in blender; blend until smooth.

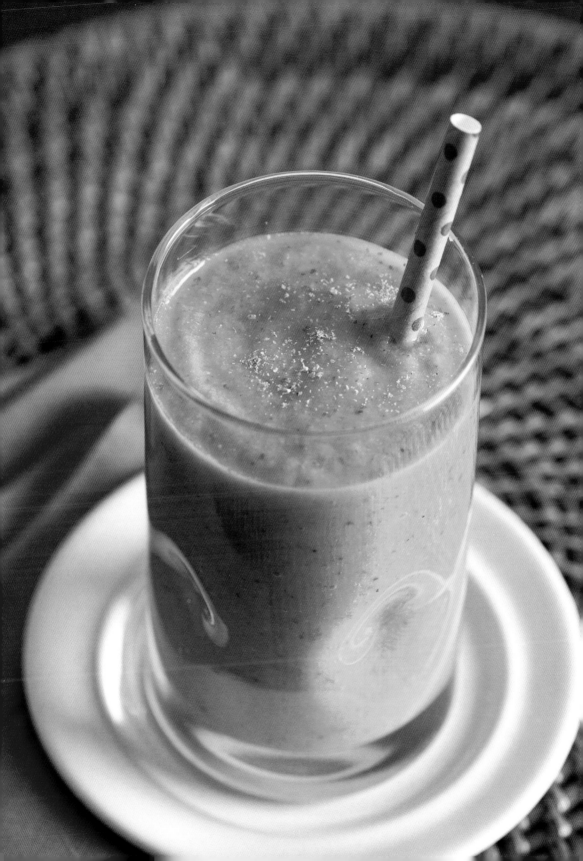

GREEN PINEAPPLE PICK-ME-UP

MAKES 1 SERVING

½ cup frozen pineapple chunks

½ avocado, pitted and peeled

1 cup baby kale

2 tablespoons water

1 tablespoon lime juice

1 teaspoon honey

Combine pineapple, avocado, kale, water, lime juice and honey in blender; blend until smooth.

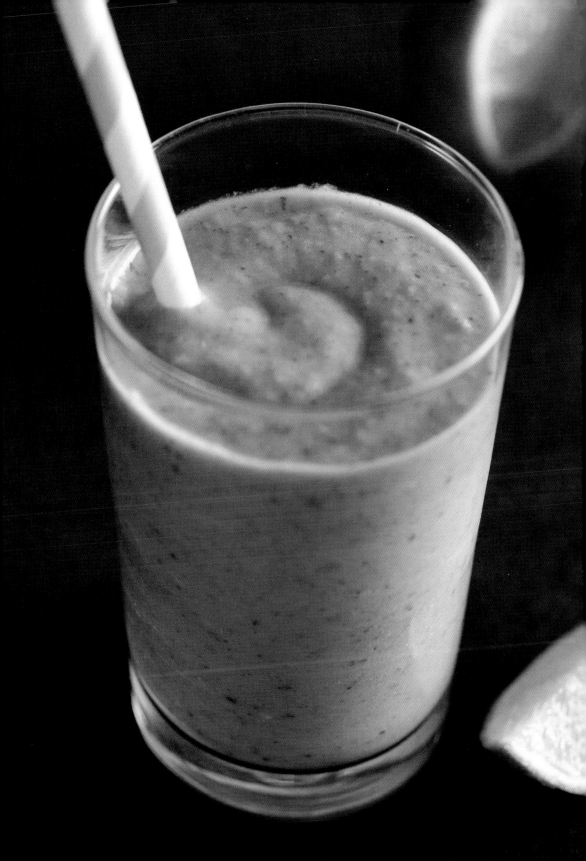

CRANBERRY APPLE CRUSH
MAKES 1 SERVING

¼ cup water

1 sweet red apple, seeded and cut into chunks

½ cup fresh or thawed frozen cranberries

½ frozen banana

2 teaspoons honey

⅛ teaspoon ground cinnamon

Combine water, apple, cranberries, banana, honey and cinnamon in blender; blend until smooth.

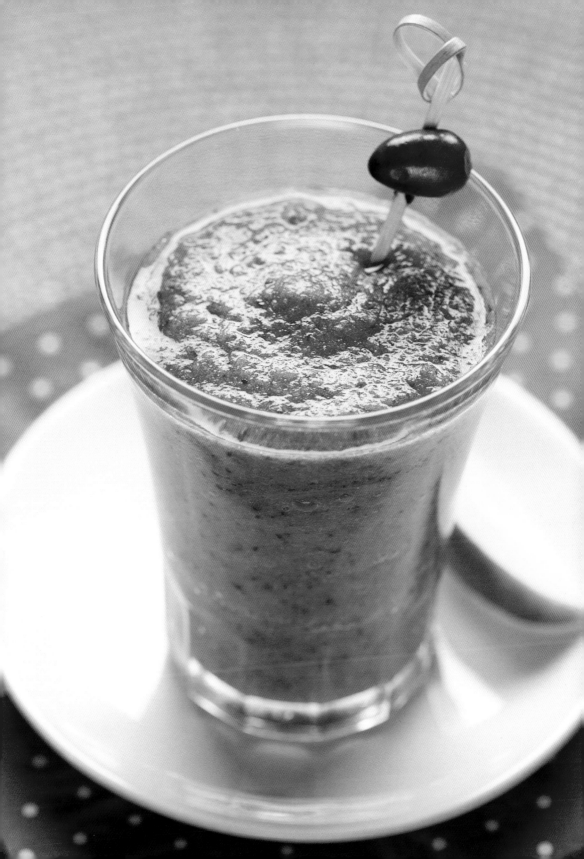

RAPID REFRESHERS

....

RASPBERRY PEAR REFRESHER
MAKES 2 SERVINGS

¾ cup water

1 pear, seeded and cut into chunks

1 clementine, peeled

1 cup frozen raspberries

Combine water, pear, clementine and raspberries in blender; blend until smooth.

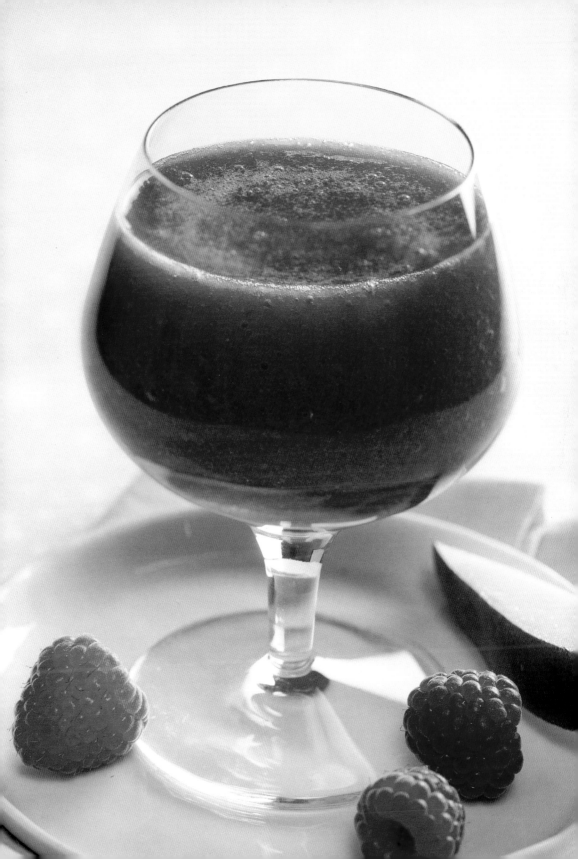

CREAMY MANGO SMOOTHIE
MAKES 3 SERVINGS

1½ **cups unsweetened coconut milk**

2 **cups frozen mango chunks**

1 **navel orange, peeled and seeded**

¾ **teaspoon vanilla**

Combine coconut milk, mango, orange and vanilla in blender; blend until smooth.

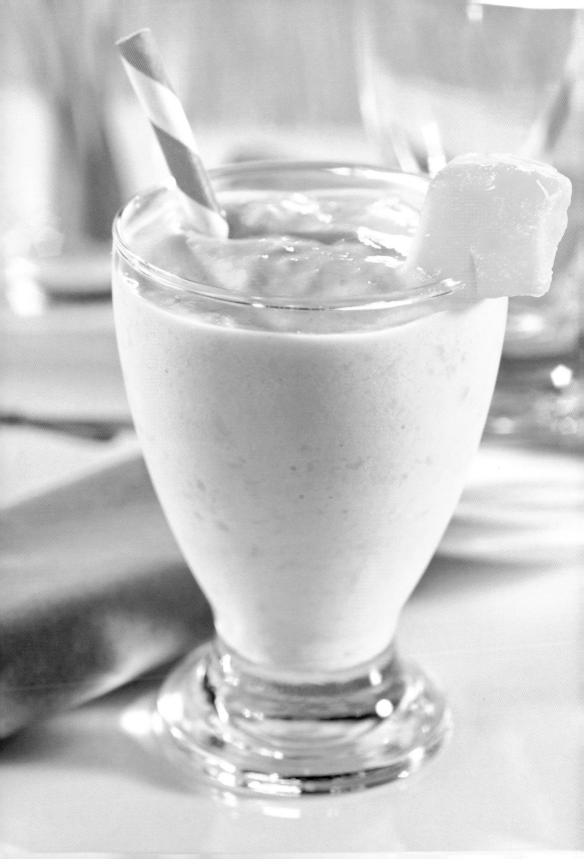

GRAPE CHERRY SMOOTHIE
MAKES 2 SERVINGS

1 cup seedless red grapes

1 navel orange, peeled and seeded

½ cup frozen dark sweet cherries

¼ cup ice cubes

Combine grapes, orange, cherries and ice in blender; blend until smooth.

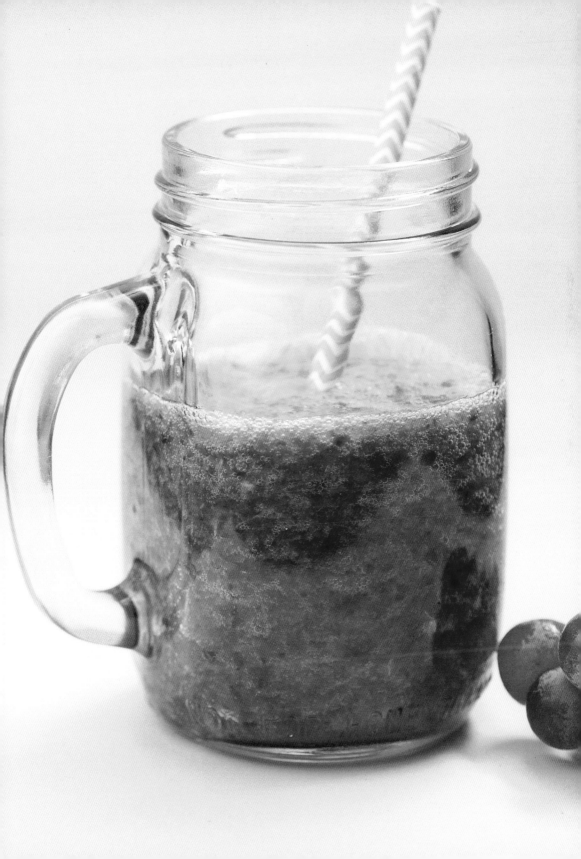

SPEEDY RASPBERRY SMOOTHIE >
MAKES 2 SERVINGS

1 cup unsweetened almond milk

2 cups frozen raspberries

½ avocado, pitted and peeled

2 tablespoons lemon juice

1 tablespoon honey

Combine almond milk, raspberries, avocado, lemon juice and honey in blender; blend until smooth.

MANGOLICIOUS BANANA SMOOTHIE
MAKES 2 SERVINGS

1 cup orange juice

1¼ cups frozen mango chunks

1 banana

Combine orange juice, mango and banana in blender; blend until smooth.

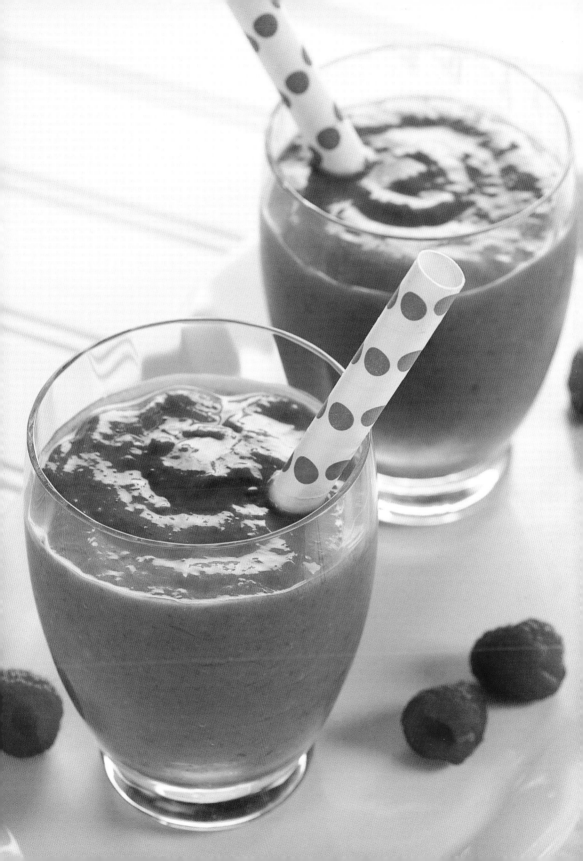

LEMON-LIME WATERMELON AGUA FRESCA
MAKES 3 SERVINGS

5 cups seedless watermelon chunks

½ cup ice water

Grated peel and juice of 1 lemon

Grated peel and juice of 1 lime

1 Combine watermelon, water, lemon peel and juice and lime peel and juice in blender; blend until smooth.

2 Serve immediately over ice or refrigerate until ready to serve.

CHOCOLATE RASPBERRY SMOOTHIE
MAKES 1 SERVING

½ cup unsweetened almond milk

1 cup frozen raspberries

1 tablespoon unsweetened cocoa powder

1 teaspoon honey

Combine almond milk, raspberries, cocoa and honey in blender; blend until smooth.

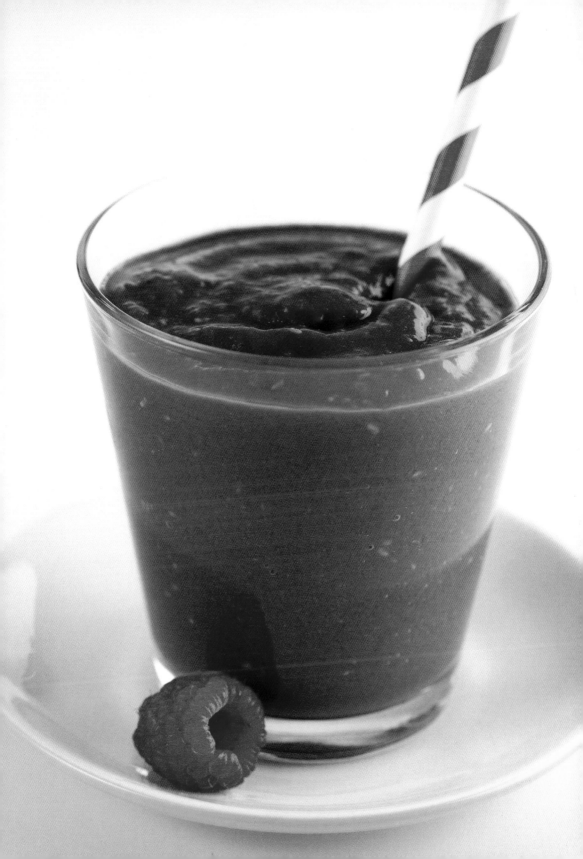

PLUM CHERRY SMOOTHIE
MAKES 1 SERVING

1 plum, pitted and cut into chunks

1 cup frozen dark sweet cherries

½ frozen banana

Combine plum, cherries and banana in blender; blend until smooth. Serve immediately.

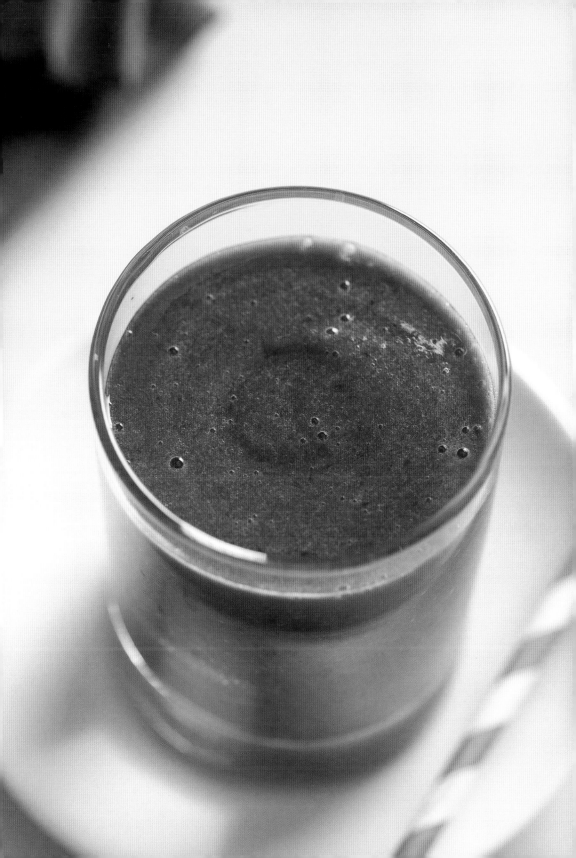

STRAWBERRY CLEMENTINE SMOOTHIE >

MAKES 2 SERVINGS

⅓ cup water

2 cups frozen strawberries, slightly thawed

1 frozen banana

2 clementines, peeled

Combine water, strawberries, banana and clementines in blender; blend until smooth.

PALEO PEACH COCONUT SMOOTHIE

MAKES 2 SERVINGS

1 cup unsweetened coconut milk

1½ cups frozen sliced peaches

¼ teaspoon grated lemon peel

Combine coconut milk, peaches and lemon peel in blender; blend until smooth.

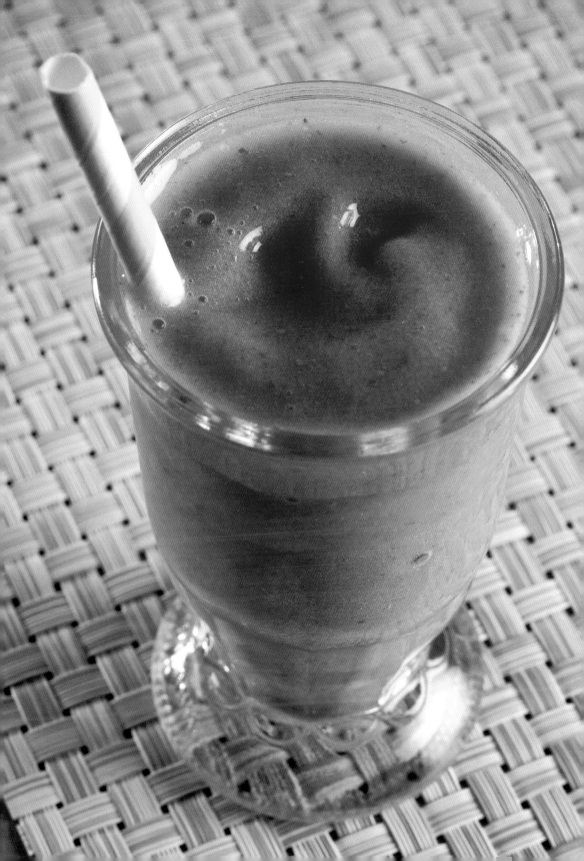

RASPBERRY CHERRY SMOOTHIE

MAKES 2 SERVINGS

⅔ cup apple juice

1 cup frozen raspberries

1 cup frozen dark sweet cherries, slightly thawed

½ avocado, pitted and peeled

Combine apple juice, raspberries, cherries and avocado in blender; blend until smooth.

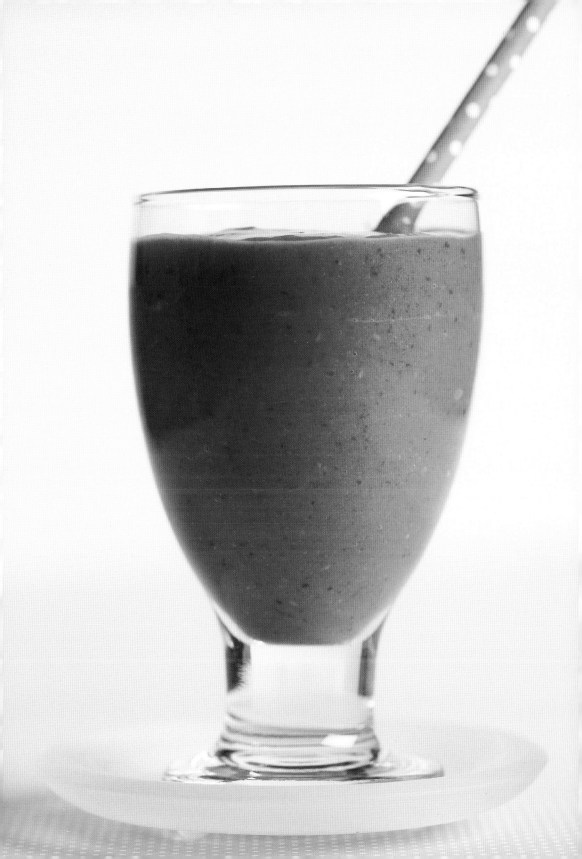

PEACH VANILLA SMOOTHIE
MAKES 1 SERVING

½ cup unsweetened almond milk

1 cup frozen sliced peaches

½ cup ice cubes

2 teaspoons honey

½ teaspoon vanilla

Combine almond milk, peaches, ice, honey and vanilla in blender; blend until smooth.

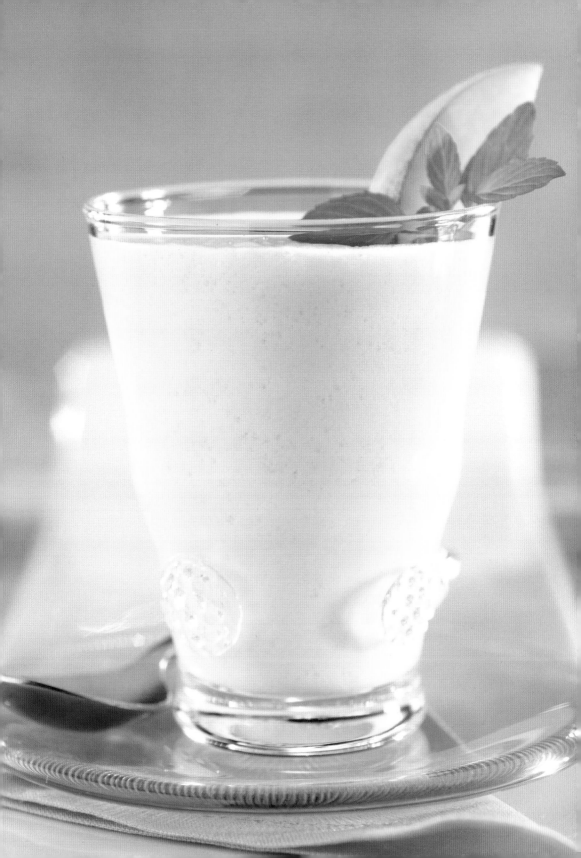

MORNING JUICES

SWEET AND SOUR
MAKES 2 SERVINGS

1½ cups fresh raspberries

⅛ papaya

½ grapefruit, peeled

Juice raspberries, papaya and grapefruit. Stir.

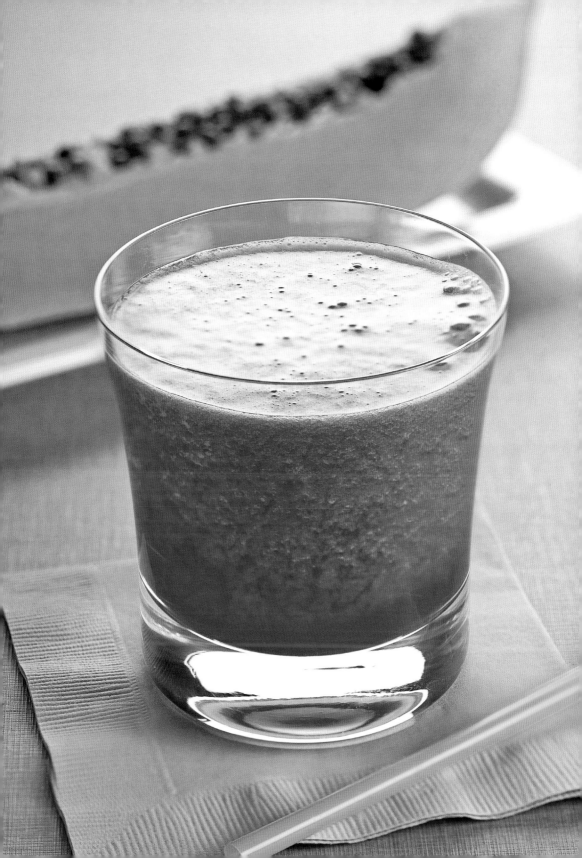

CITRUS CARROT >
MAKES 2 SERVINGS

1 orange, peeled

2 carrots

½ lemon, peeled

Juice orange, carrots and lemon. Stir.

STRAWBERRY MELON
MAKES 2 SERVINGS

½ cantaloupe, rind removed

1 cup fresh strawberries

Juice cantaloupe and strawberries. Stir.

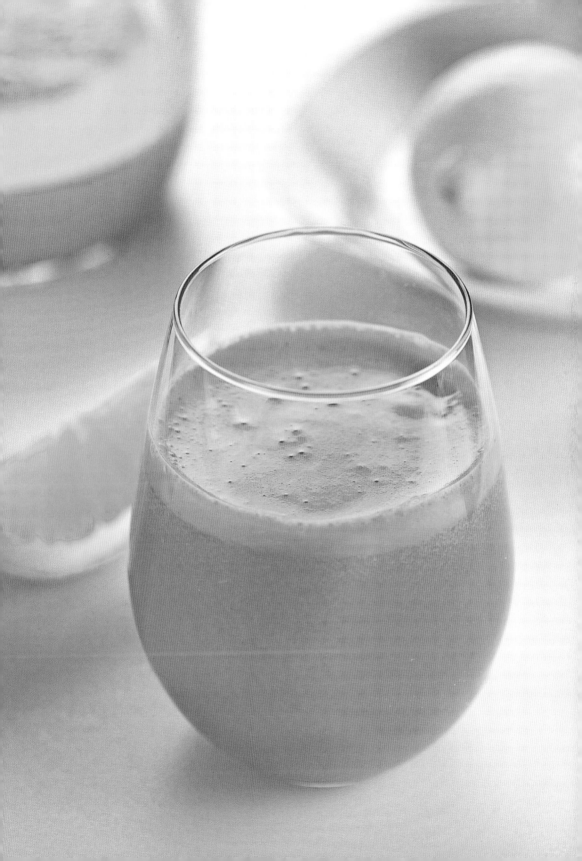

SPICY-SWEET GRAPEFRUIT >

MAKES 3 SERVINGS

2 grapefruits, peeled

5 carrots

1 inch fresh ginger, peeled

Juice grapefruits, carrots and ginger. Stir.

ORANGE TRIPLE THREAT

MAKES 3 SERVINGS

8 carrots

1 mango, peeled

1 orange, peeled

Juice carrots, mango and orange. Stir.

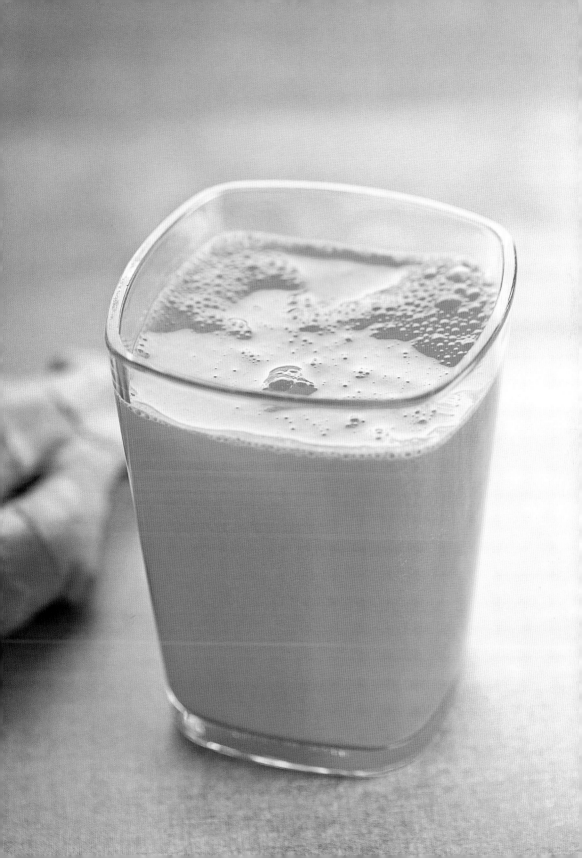

MELON REFRESHER >
MAKES 2 SERVINGS

¼ cantaloupe, rind removed

1 pear

1 lime, peeled

2 sprigs fresh mint

Juice cantaloupe, pear, lime and mint. Stir.

CITRUS BLUSH
MAKES 2 SERVINGS

1 grapefruit, peeled

1 peach

1 apple

Juice grapefruit, peach and apple. Stir.

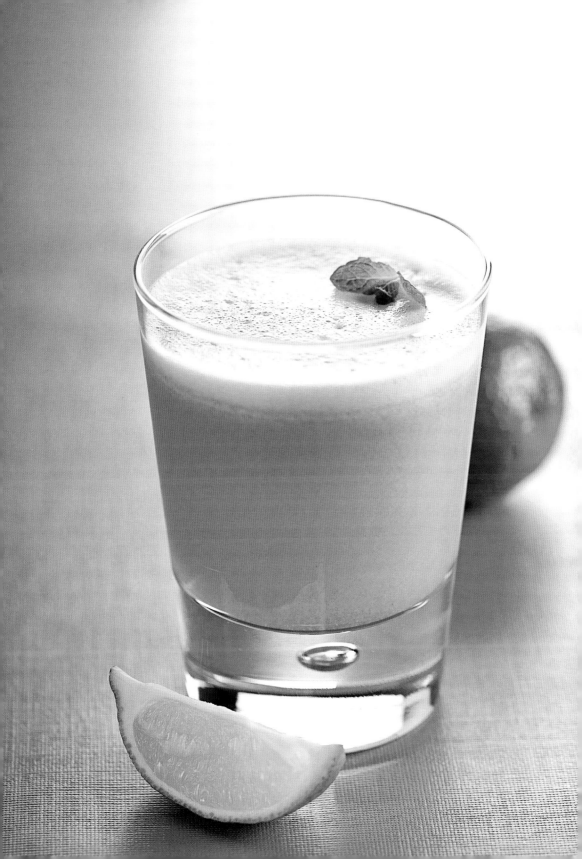

ISLAND ORANGE JUICE >

MAKES 2 SERVINGS

2 oranges, peeled

2 guavas

½ cup fresh strawberries

Juice oranges, guavas and strawberries. Stir.

WORKOUT WARMUP

MAKES 2 SERVINGS

2 apples

2 kiwis, peeled

½ cup fresh strawberries

4 leaves kale

½ lime, peeled

Juice apples, kiwis, strawberries, kale and lime. Stir.

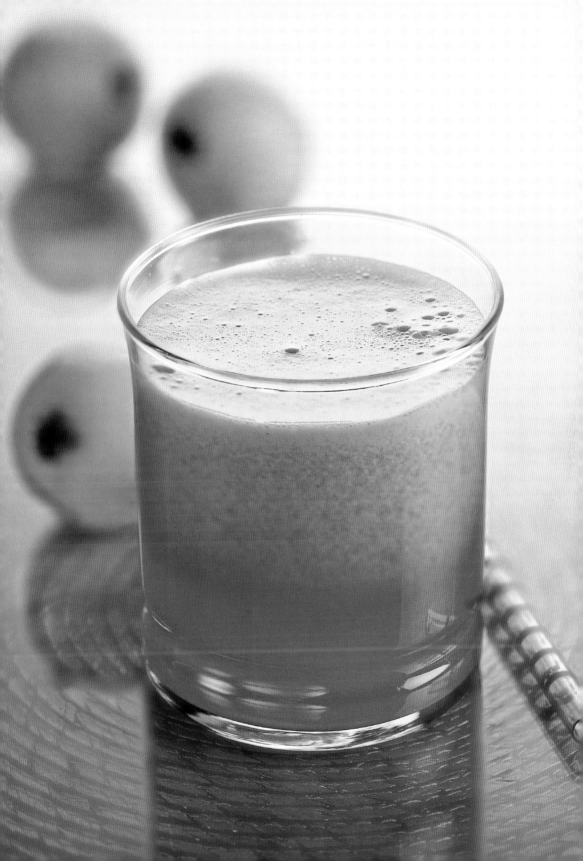

TANGERINE APPLE JUICE >
MAKES 2 SERVINGS

2 apples

2 tangerines, peeled

¼ lemon, peeled

Juice apples, tangerines and lemon. Stir.

EARLY RISER BREAKFAST
MAKES 2 SERVINGS

1 beet

¼ red cabbage

2 carrots

½ red bell pepper

1 orange, peeled

1 apple

½ lemon, peeled

Juice beet, cabbage, carrots, bell pepper, orange, apple and lemon. Stir.

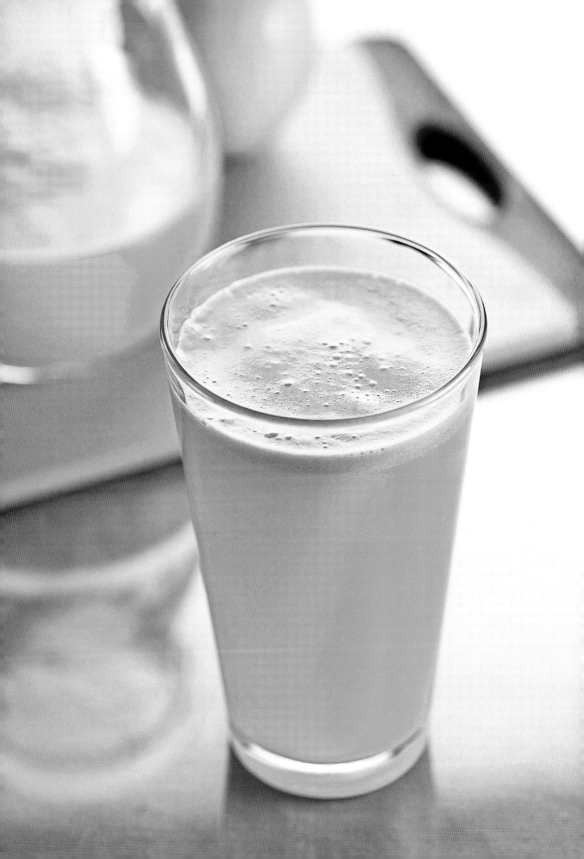

RED ORANGE JUICE >

MAKES 2 SERVINGS

1 orange, peeled
1 apple
½ cup fresh raspberries
½ cup fresh strawberries

Juice orange, apple, raspberries and strawberries. Stir.

BLUEBERRY HAZE

MAKES 2 SERVINGS

2 apples
1½ cups fresh blueberries
½ grapefruit, peeled
1 inch fresh ginger, peeled

Juice apples, blueberries, grapefruit and ginger. Stir.

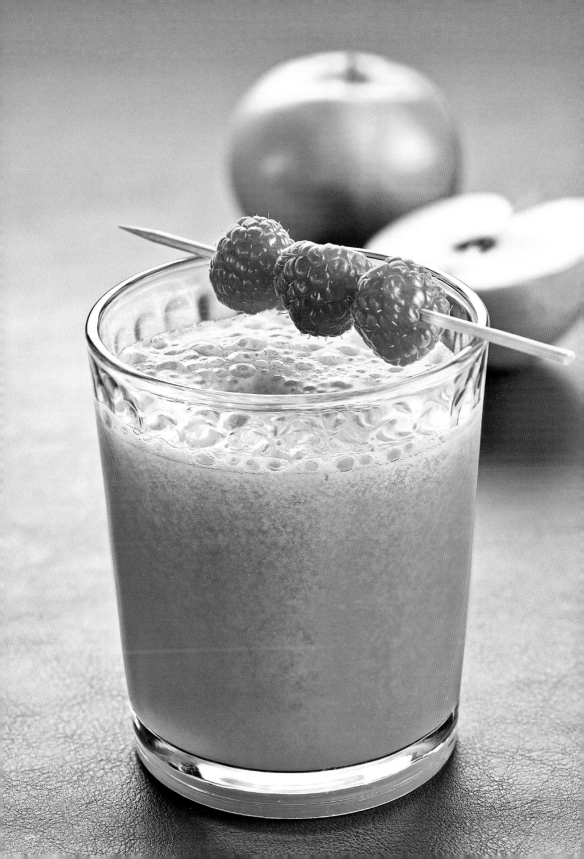

POMEGRANATE APPLE >
MAKES 2 SERVINGS

2 pomegranates, peeled

2 apples

Juice pomegranate seeds and apples. Stir.

TRIPLE GREEN
MAKES 2 SERVINGS

½ honeydew melon, rind removed

1 cucumber

4 leaves kale

Juice honeydew, cucumber and kale. Stir.

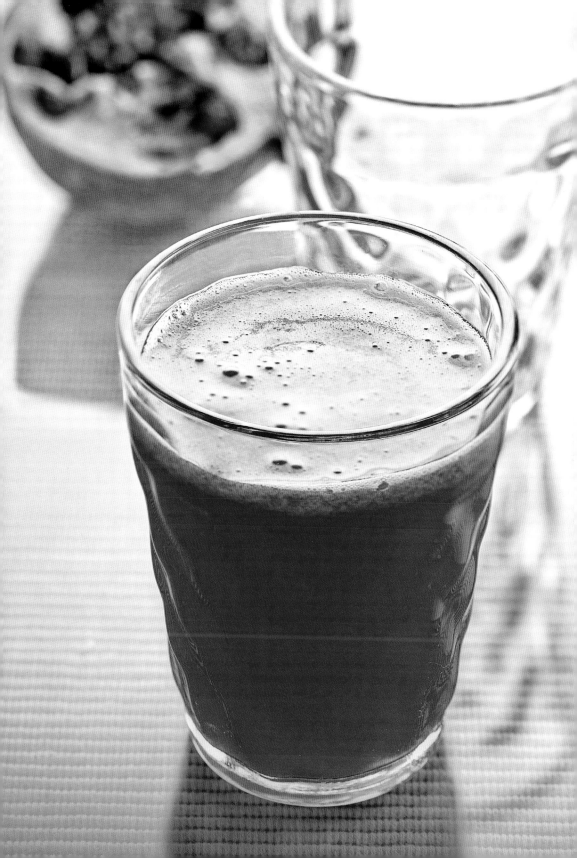

SUNSET BERRY >

1 cup fresh strawberries

1 orange, peeled

½ lime, peeled

Juice strawberries, orange and lime. Stir.

TROPICAL TWIST

MAKES 2 SERVINGS

⅛ pineapple, peeled

⅛ seedless watermelon, rind removed

1 orange, peeled

½ mango, peeled

⅓ cup fresh strawberries

Juice pineapple, watermelon, orange, mango and strawberries. Stir.

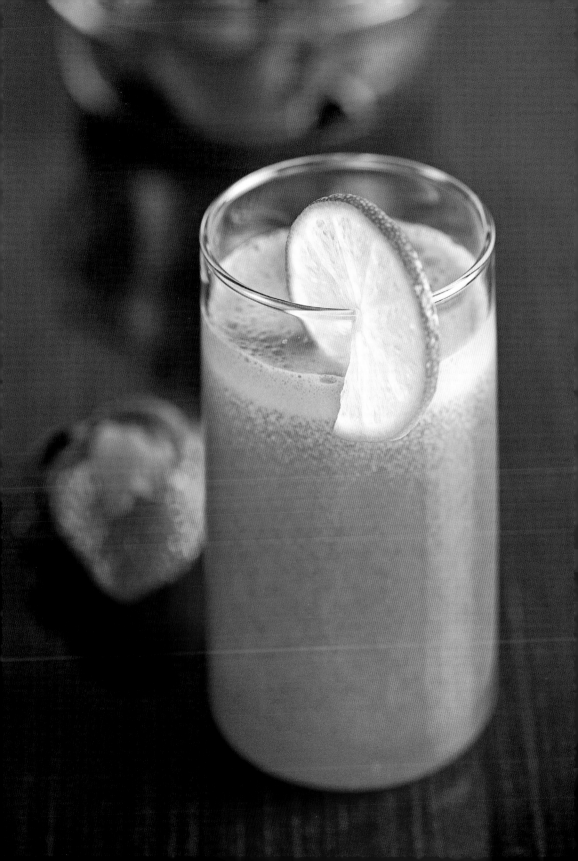

HEALTHY ELIXIRS

··

COLD AND FLU NINJA JUICE
MAKES 1 SERVING

1 orange, peeled
½ lemon, peeled
⅛ small red onion
1 clove garlic
½ teaspoon honey

Juice orange, lemon, onion and garlic. Stir in honey until well blended.

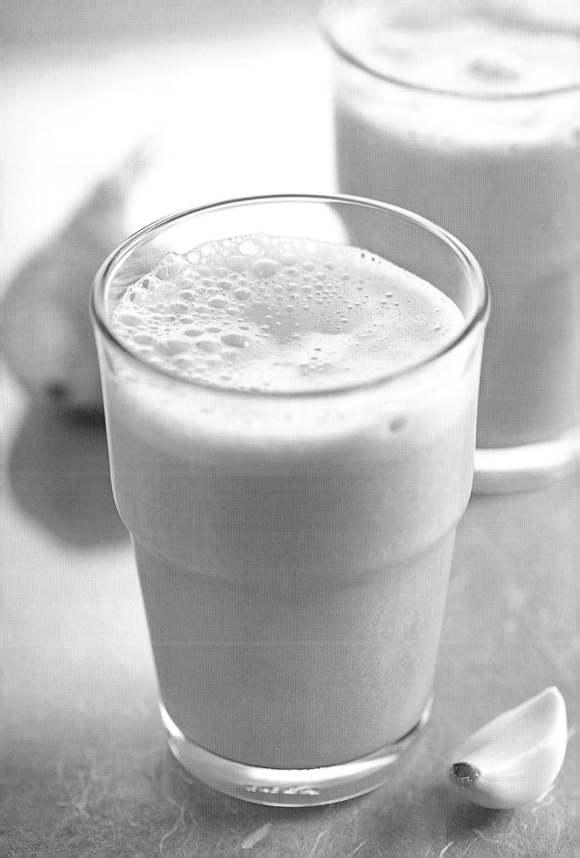

CRANBERRY PEAR BLAST >

MAKES 2 SERVINGS

2 pears

½ cucumber

¾ cup fresh or thawed frozen cranberries

¼ lemon, peeled

½ to 1 inch fresh ginger, peeled

Juice pears, cucumber, cranberries, lemon and ginger. Stir.

VITAMIN BOOST

MAKES 2 SERVINGS

¼ cantaloupe, rind removed

1 orange, peeled

¼ papaya

2 leaves Swiss chard

Juice cantaloupe, orange, papaya and chard. Stir.

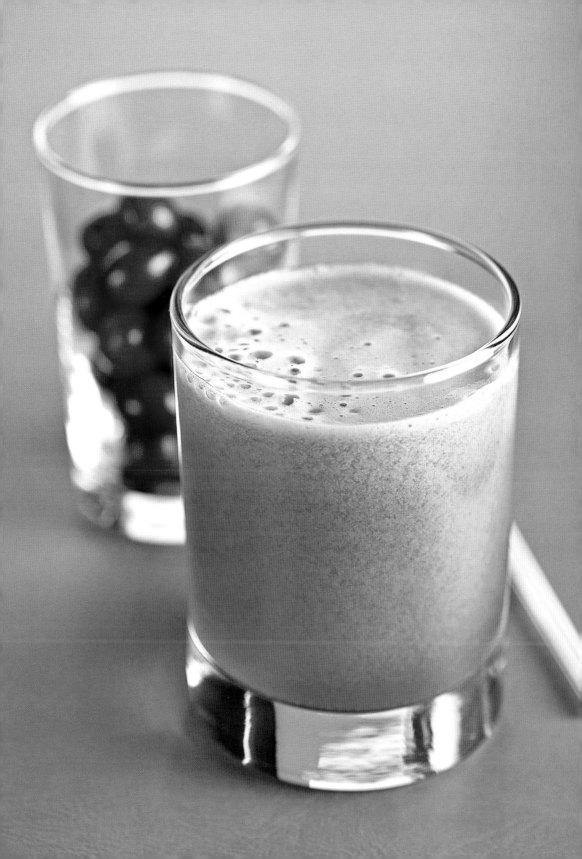

GREEN ENERGY >

MAKES 4 SERVINGS

- 2 stalks celery
- 2 apples
- 6 leaves kale
- ½ cup packed spinach
- ½ cucumber
- ¼ bulb fennel
- ½ lemon, peeled
- 1 inch fresh ginger, peeled

Juice celery, apples, kale, spinach, cucumber, fennel, lemon and ginger. Stir.

BETA-CAROTENE BLAST

MAKES 2 SERVINGS

- 4 carrots
- 1 apple
- 4 leaves bok choy
- 2 leaves kale
- ½ inch fresh ginger, peeled

Juice carrots, apple, bok choy, kale and ginger. Stir.

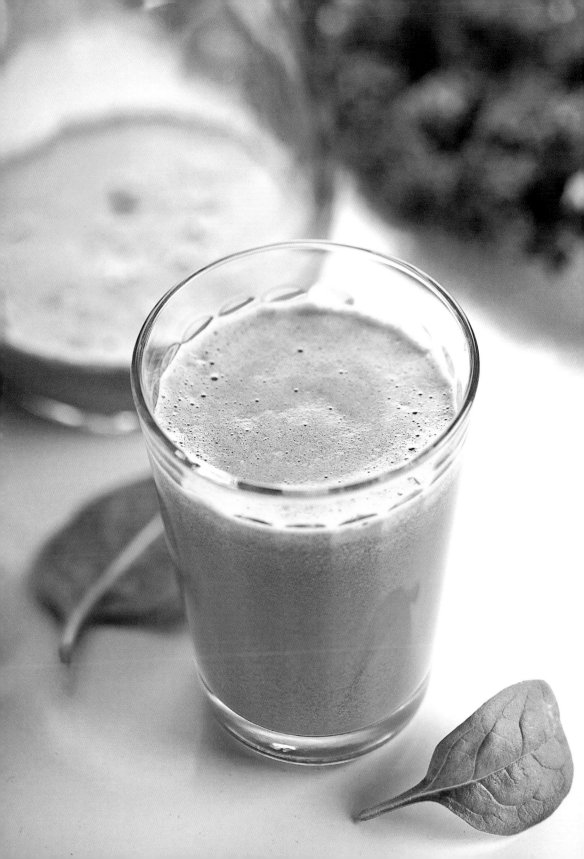

HEADACHE BUSTER >
MAKES 1 SERVING

1 cup cauliflower florets

1 cup broccoli florets

1 apple

Juice cauliflower, broccoli and apple. Stir.

CHERRY GREEN JUICE
MAKES 2 SERVINGS

1 cup fresh cherries, pitted

2 stalks celery

1 apple

1 cup fresh parsley

1 lemon, peeled

Juice cherries, celery, apple, parsley and lemon. Stir.

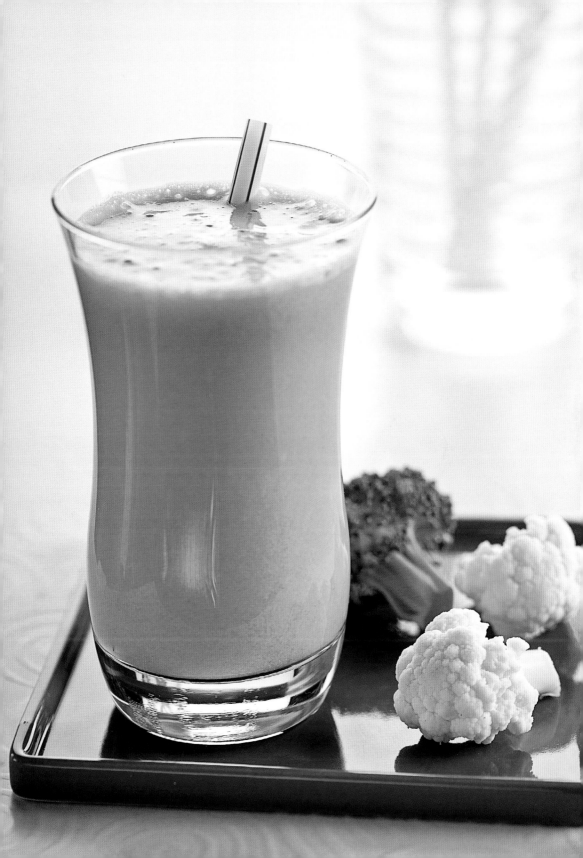

ANTIOXIDANT COCKTAIL >

MAKES 3 SERVINGS

1 grapefruit, peeled

2 oranges, peeled

½ cup fresh blackberries

Juice grapefruit, oranges and blackberries. Stir.

HONEY SPICE

MAKES 2 SERVINGS

1 grapefruit, peeled

¼ pineapple, peeled

½ inch fresh ginger, peeled

4 whole cloves

1 teaspoon honey

1 Juice grapefruit, pineapple and ginger. Stir.

2 Pour juice mixture into medium saucepan. Add cloves and honey; simmer over low heat until heated through. Remove from heat; set aside 5 minutes. Strain.

HEALTHY ELIXIRS

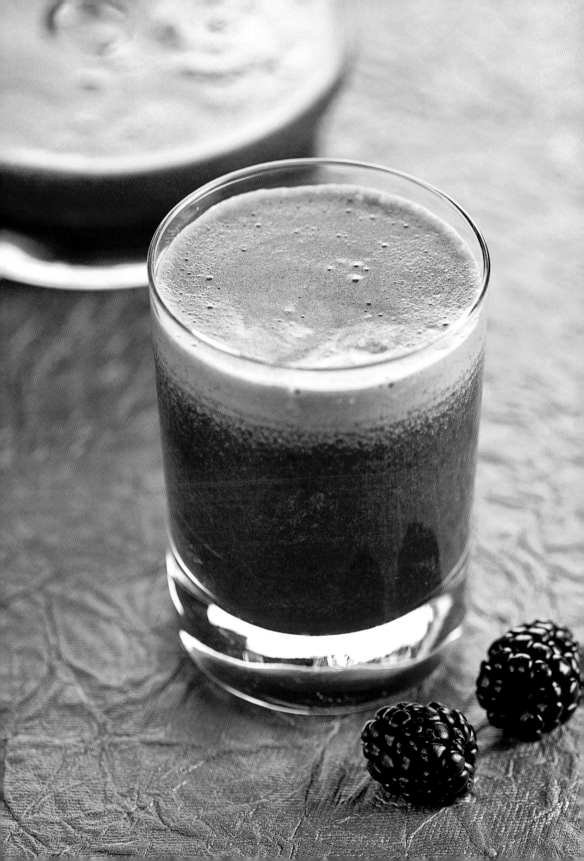

JOINT COMFORT JUICE >

MAKES 2 SERVINGS

2 cups packed spinach

¼ pineapple, peeled

1 pear

1 cup fresh parsley

½ grapefruit, peeled

Juice spinach, pineapple, pear, parsley and grapefruit. Stir.

KALE-APPLE-CARROT

MAKES 2 SERVINGS

3 carrots

2 stalks celery

1 apple

3 leaves kale

½ cup fresh parsley

Juice carrots, celery, apple, kale and parsley. Stir.

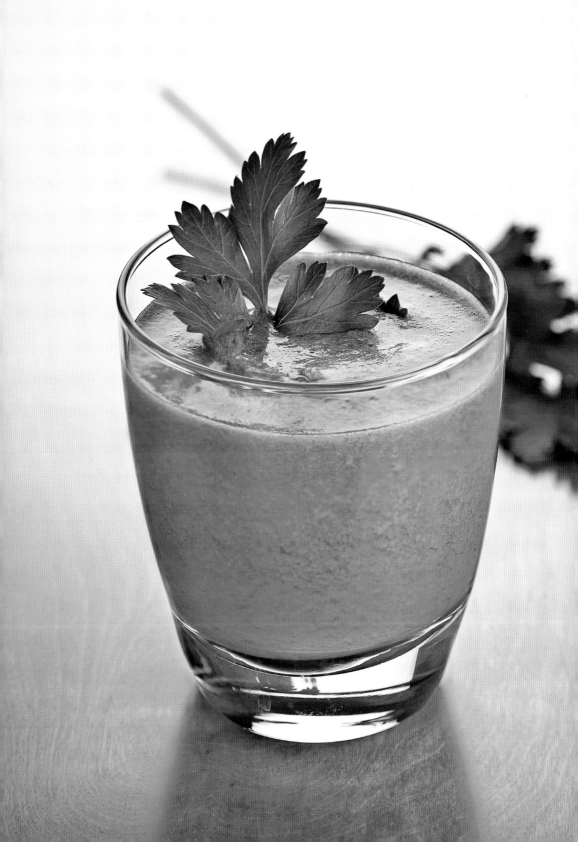

PLUM CHERRY >
MAKES 2 SERVINGS

2 dark plums

1½ cups fresh cherries, pitted

Juice plums and cherries. Stir.

MINT JULEP JUICE
MAKES 1 SERVING

1 apple

1 cup packed spinach

1 stalk celery

1 cup fresh mint

Juice apple, spinach, celery and mint. Stir.

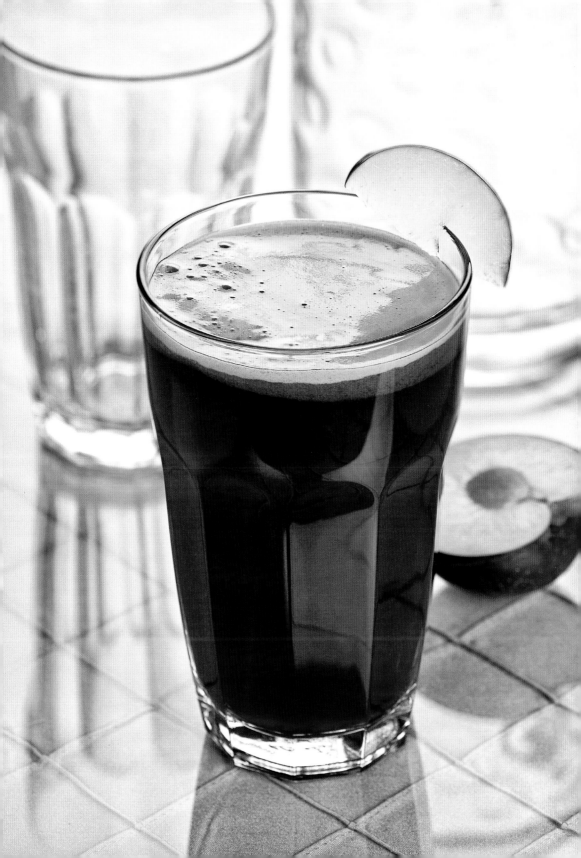

CLEANSING GREEN JUICE >

MAKES 2 SERVINGS

4 leaves bok choy

1 stalk celery

½ cucumber

¼ bulb fennel

½ lemon, peeled

Juice bok choy, celery, cucumber, fennel and lemon. Stir.

PURPLEBERRY JUICE

MAKES 2 SERVINGS

2 cups red seedless grapes

1 apple

½ cup fresh blackberries

½ inch fresh ginger, peeled

Juice grapes, apple, blackberries and ginger. Stir.

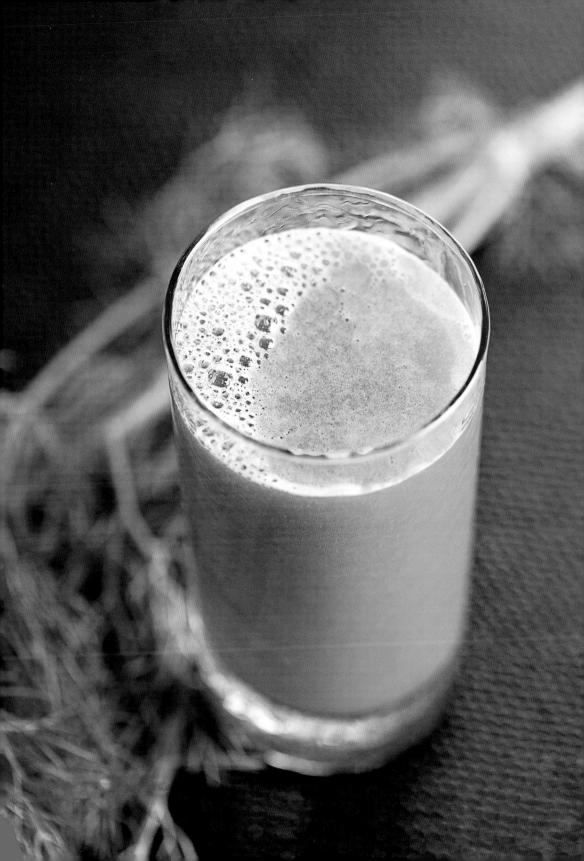

POMEGRANATE-LIME-COCONUT JUICE >
MAKES 2 SERVINGS

1 pomegranate, peeled

½ cucumber

1 lime, peeled

¼ cup coconut water

Juice pomegranate seeds, cucumber and lime. Stir in coconut water until well blended.

PAPAYA POWER JUICE
MAKES 2 SERVINGS

¼ papaya

1 orange, peeled

¾ cup fresh parsley

1 clove garlic

Juice papaya, orange, parsley and garlic. Stir.

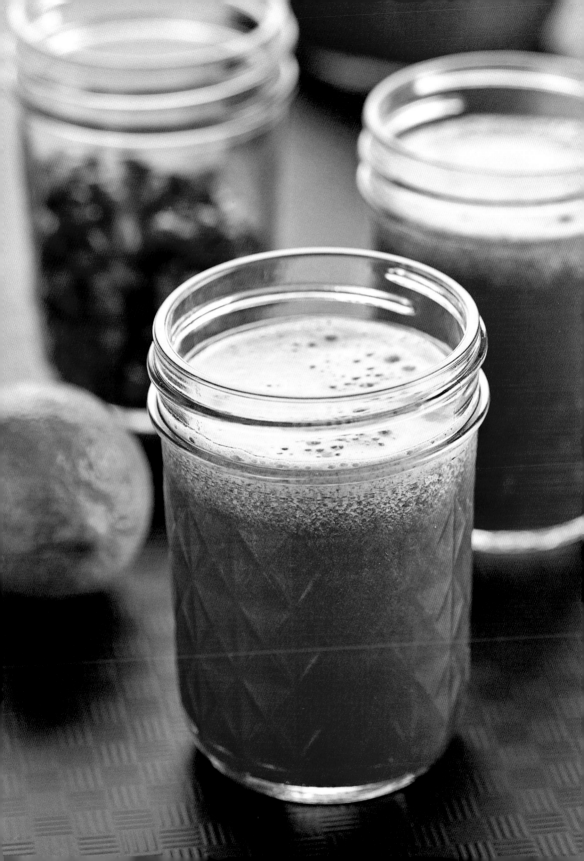

CITRUS SPROUT >
MAKES 2 SERVINGS

1 cup brussels sprouts

4 leaves romaine lettuce

1 orange, peeled

½ apple

½ lemon, peeled

Juice brussels sprouts, romaine, orange, apple and lemon. Stir.

SUPER BERRY REFRESHER
MAKES 2 SERVINGS

1 cup fresh strawberries

1 cup fresh raspberries

1 cucumber

½ cup fresh blackberries

½ cup fresh blueberries

¼ lemon, peeled

Juice strawberries, raspberries, cucumber, blackberries, blueberries and lemon. Stir.

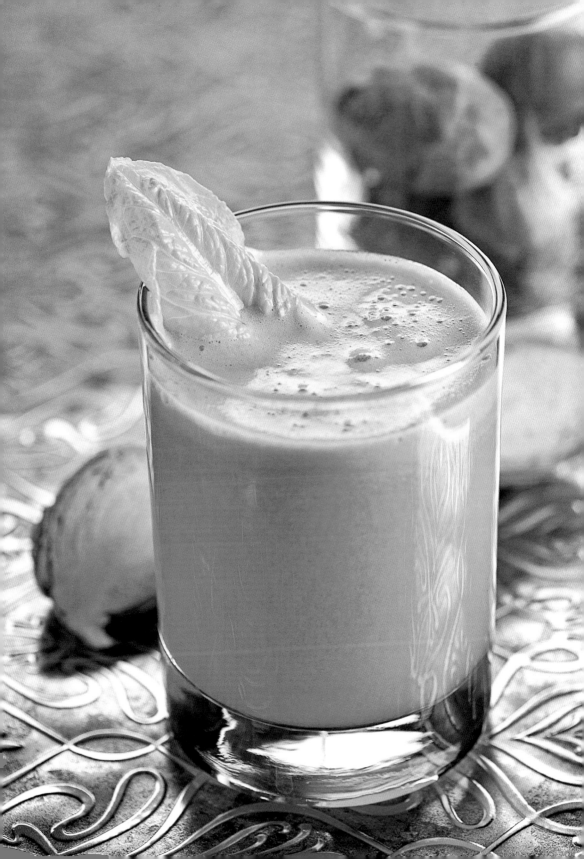

REFRESHING ROOTS

· ·

APPLE, TATER AND CARROT
MAKES 4 SERVINGS

4 apples
1 sweet potato
1 carrot

Juice apples, sweet potato and carrot. Stir.

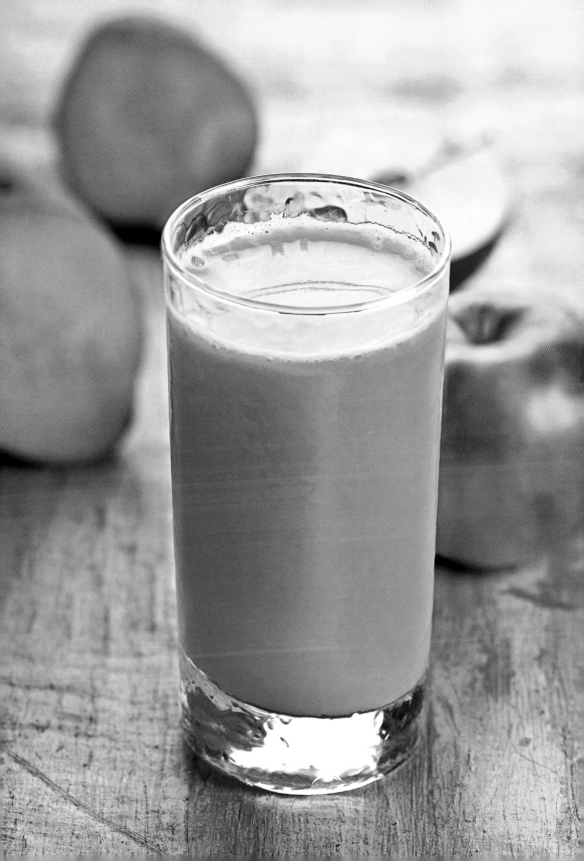

RUBY APPLE STINGER >

2 beets

2 carrots

½ apple

1 inch fresh ginger, peeled

¼ lemon, peeled

Juice beets, carrots, apple, ginger and lemon. Stir.

ROOTY TOOTY

MAKES 2 SERVINGS

2 carrots

4 radishes

1 cup fresh parsley

½ cup cut-up peeled rutabaga

Juice carrots, radishes, parsley and rutabaga. Stir.

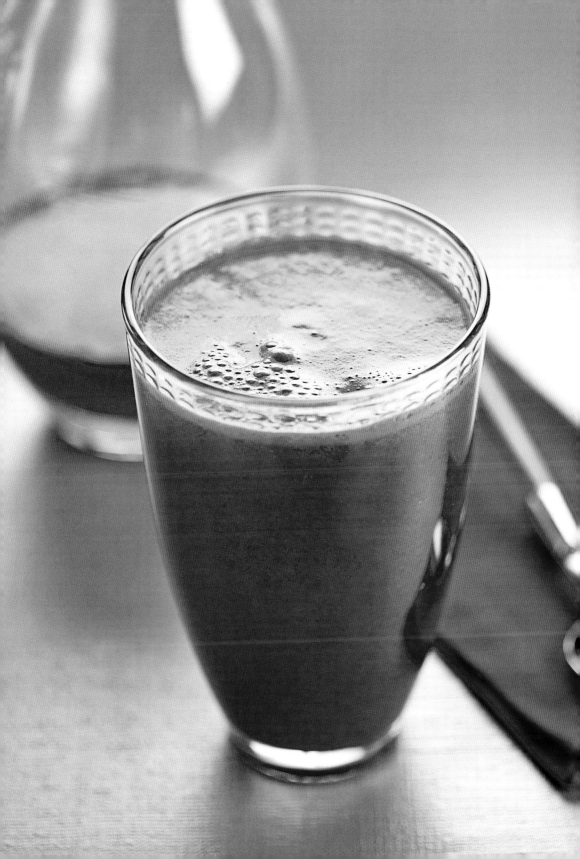

EASY BEING GREEN >

MAKES 2 SERVINGS

2 cups watercress

2 parsnips

2 stalks celery

½ cucumber

4 sprigs fresh basil

Juice watercress, parsnips, celery, cucumber and basil. Stir.

CELERY ROOT-BEET-CARROT JUICE

MAKES 2 SERVINGS

4 carrots

1 apple

1 beet

½ celery root, peeled

¼ inch fresh ginger, peeled

Juice carrots, apple, beet, celery root and ginger. Stir.

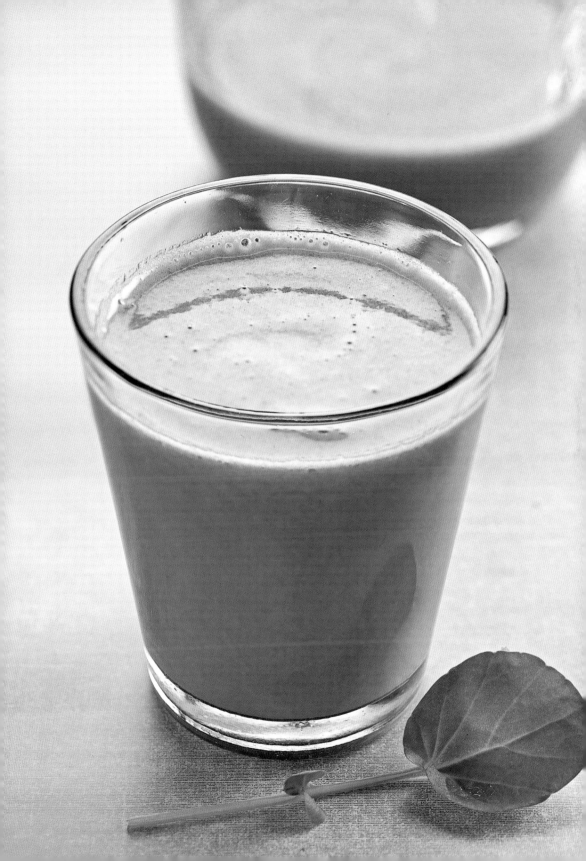

SPICY PINEAPPLE CARROT >

MAKES 2 SERVINGS

½ pineapple, peeled

2 carrots

1 inch fresh ginger, peeled

　Ice cubes

Juice pineapple, carrots and ginger. Stir. Serve over ice.

GARDEN JUICE

MAKES 2 SERVINGS

2 carrots

1 yellow bell pepper

1 apple

1 cup broccoli florets

1 beet

½ sweet potato

1 cup fresh parsley

Juice carrots, bell pepper, apple, broccoli, beet, sweet potato and parsley. Stir.

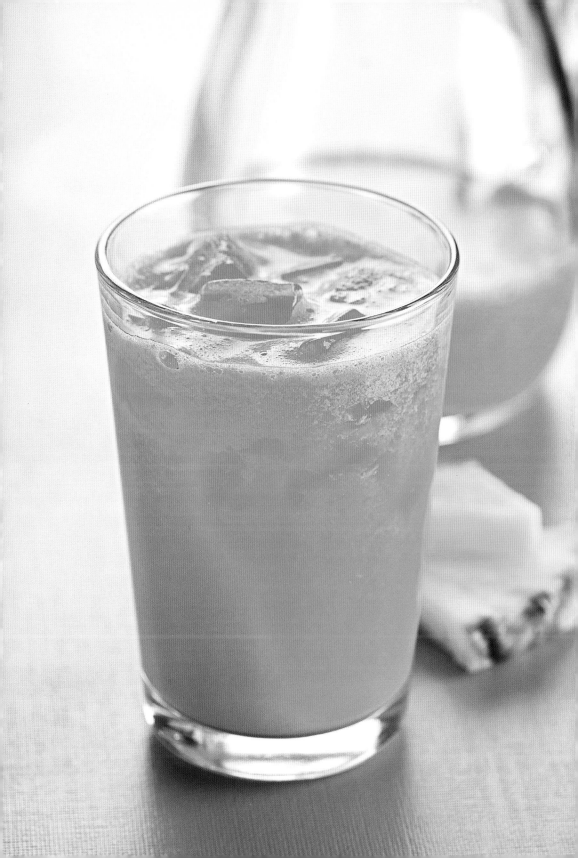

TANGY TWIST >

MAKES 3 SERVINGS

1 grapefruit, peeled

4 carrots

1 apple

1 beet

1 inch fresh ginger, peeled

Ice cubes

Juice grapefruit, carrots, apple, beet and ginger. Stir.
Serve over ice.

ORANGE BEET

MAKES 2 SERVINGS

2 oranges, peeled

1 beet

Juice oranges and beet. Stir.

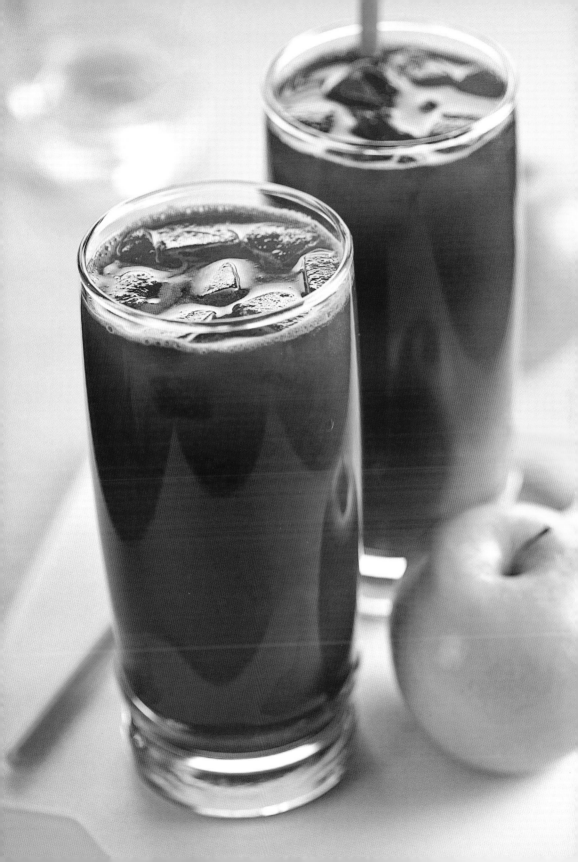

VEGGIE DELIGHT >

MAKES 2 SERVINGS

1 carrot

1 stalk celery

1 beet

1 apple

½ small sweet onion

Juice carrot, celery, beet, apple and onion. Stir.

ZIPPY PINEAPPLE CELERY

MAKES 2 SERVINGS

½ pineapple, peeled

2 radishes

1 stalk celery

Juice pineapple, radishes and celery. Stir.

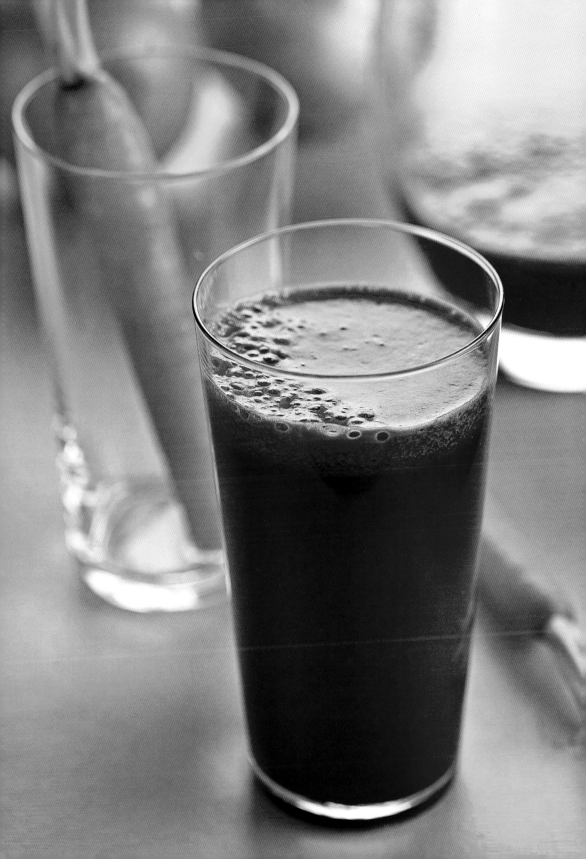

JICAMA PEAR CARROT >

MAKES 1 SERVING

　1 cup cut-up peeled jicama

½ pear

2 carrots

½ inch fresh ginger, peeled

　Pinch ground red pepper (optional)

Juice jicama, pear, carrots and ginger. Stir in red pepper, if desired, until well blended.

VEGGIE CHILLER

MAKES 2 SERVINGS

3 carrots

1 beet

½ sweet potato

¼ bulb fennel

Juice carrots, beet, sweet potato and fennel. Stir.

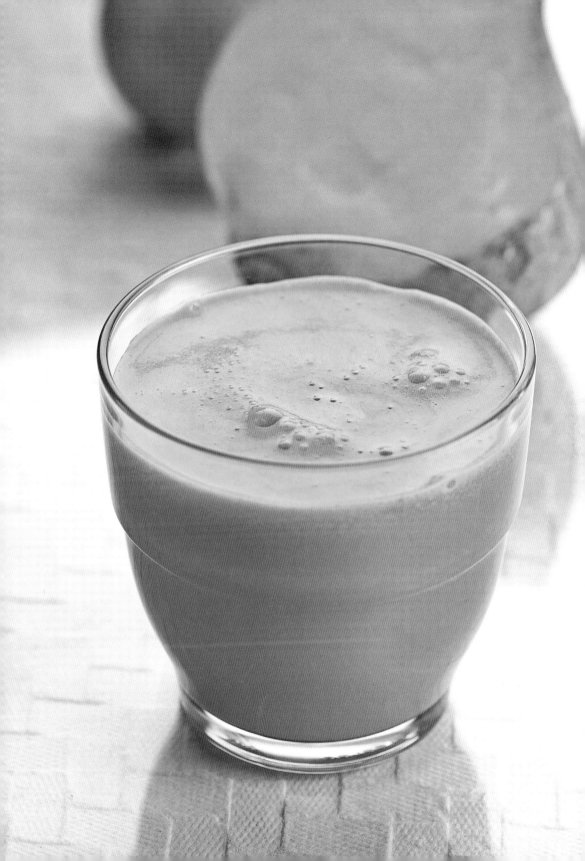

PURPLE PINEAPPLE JUICE >
MAKES 2 SERVINGS

1 beet

1 pear

¼ pineapple, peeled

1 inch fresh ginger, peeled

Juice beet, pear, pineapple and ginger. Stir.

PARSNIP PARTY
MAKES 2 SERVINGS

3 parsnips

1 apple

1 pear

½ bulb fennel

½ cup fresh parsley

Juice parsnips, apple, pear, fennel and parsley. Stir.

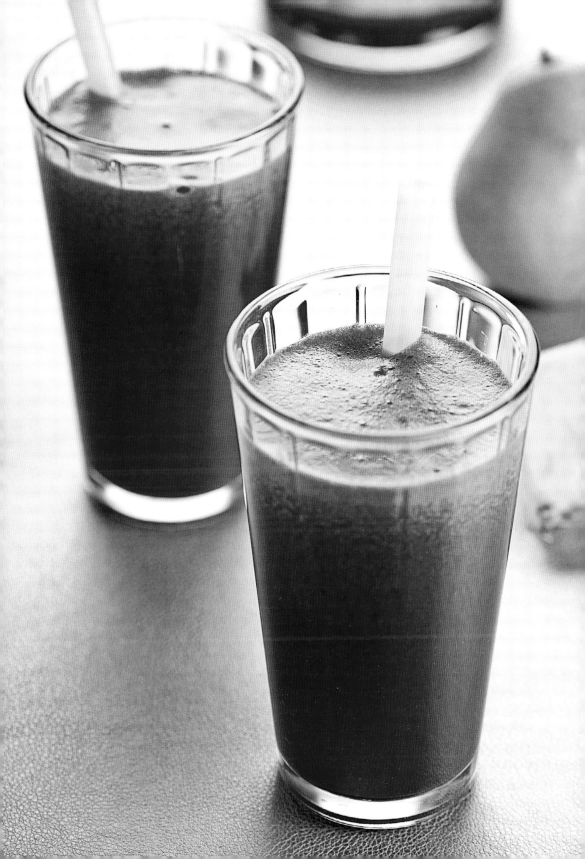

FIERY CUCUMBER BEET JUICE >
MAKES 2 SERVINGS

- 1 cucumber
- 1 beet
- 1 lemon, peeled
- 1 inch fresh ginger, peeled
- ½ jalapeño pepper

Juice cucumber, beet, lemon, ginger and jalapeño pepper. Stir.

BITE-YOU-BACK VEGGIE JUICE
MAKES 2 SERVINGS

- 3 carrots
- 1 cucumber
- 1 apple
- 2 stalks celery
- 3 leaves mustard greens

Juice carrots, cucumber, apple, celery and mustard greens. Stir.

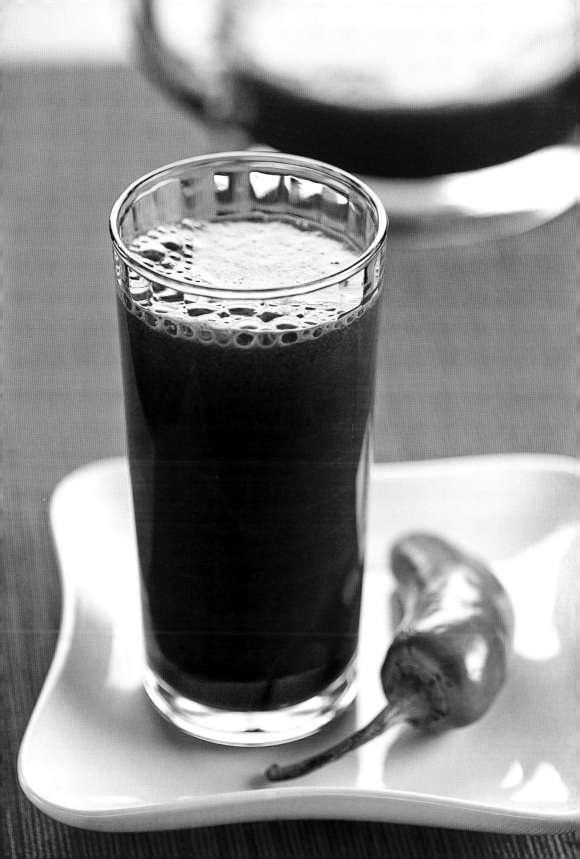

VEGETABLE VITALITY

. . . .

WALDORF JUICE

MAKES 2 SERVINGS

2 apples

6 leaves beet greens, Swiss chard or kale

2 stalks celery

Juice apples, beet greens and celery. Stir.

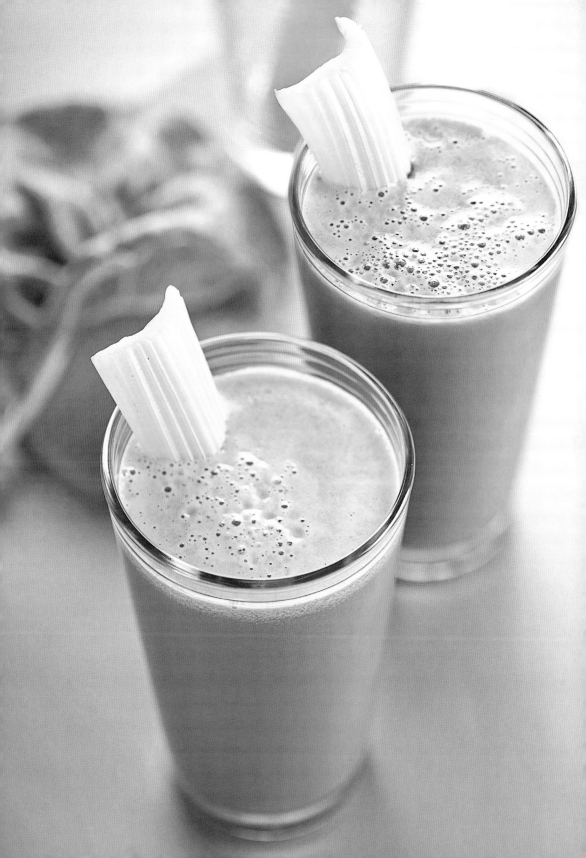

APPLE CARROT ZINGER >

MAKES 2 SERVINGS

4 carrots

2 apples

¼ cucumber

1 inch fresh ginger, peeled

Juice carrots, apples, cucumber and ginger. Stir.

RAINBOW JUICE

MAKES 2 SERVINGS

8 leaves Swiss chard

1 Asian pear

1 apple

1 beet

1 carrot

¼ head green cabbage

Juice chard, pear, apple, beet, carrot and cabbage. Stir.

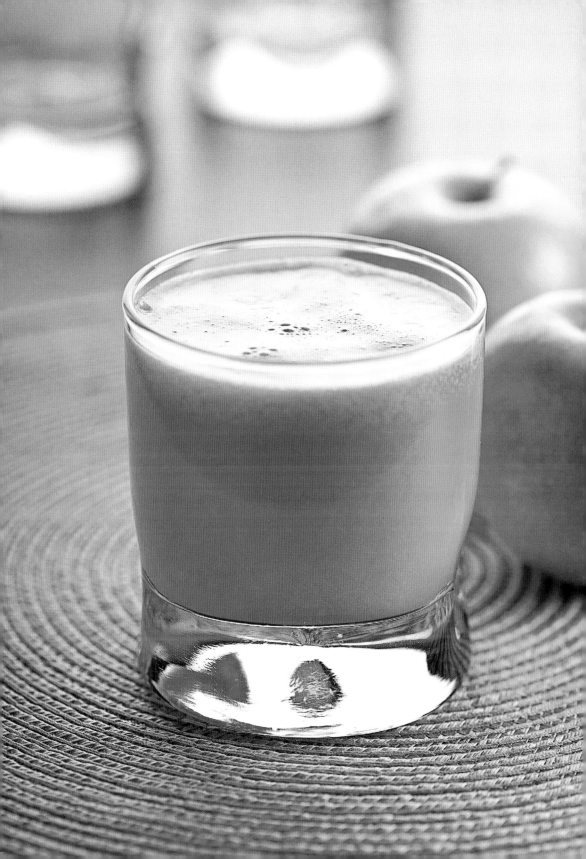

GREEN JUICE >

2 cups packed spinach

2 cucumbers

1 pear

½ lemon, peeled

1 inch fresh ginger, peeled

Juice spinach, cucumbers, pear, lemon and ginger. Stir.

SIMPLE GARDEN BLEND

MAKES 2 SERVINGS

3 carrots

2 apples

1 zucchini

Juice carrots, apples and zucchini. Stir.

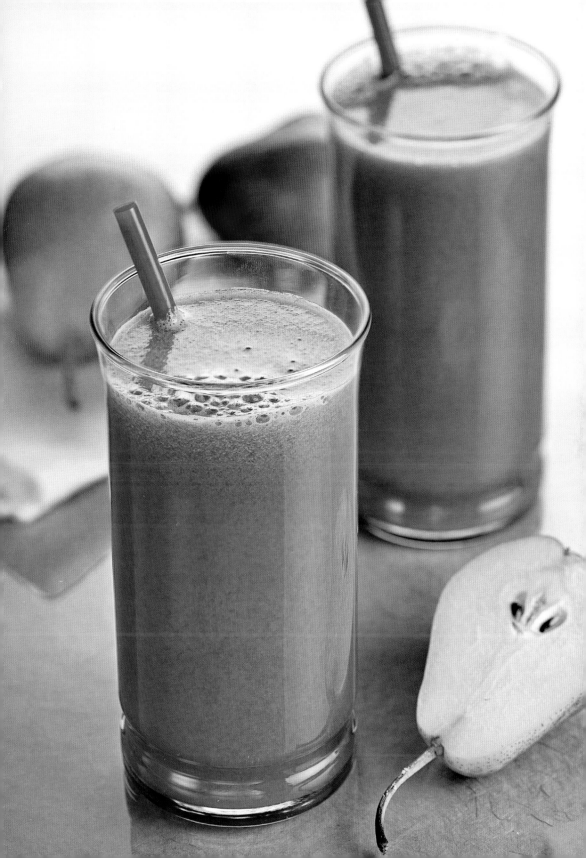

TROPICAL VEGGIE JUICE >

MAKES 2 SERVINGS

5 leaves kale

⅛ pineapple, peeled

½ cucumber

½ cup coconut water

Juice kale, pineapple and cucumber. Stir in coconut water until well blended.

CRIMSON CARROT

MAKES 2 SERVINGS

½ red cabbage

2 apples

1 carrot

⅓ cup red seedless grapes

Ice cubes

Juice cabbage, apple, carrot and grapes. Stir. Serve over ice.

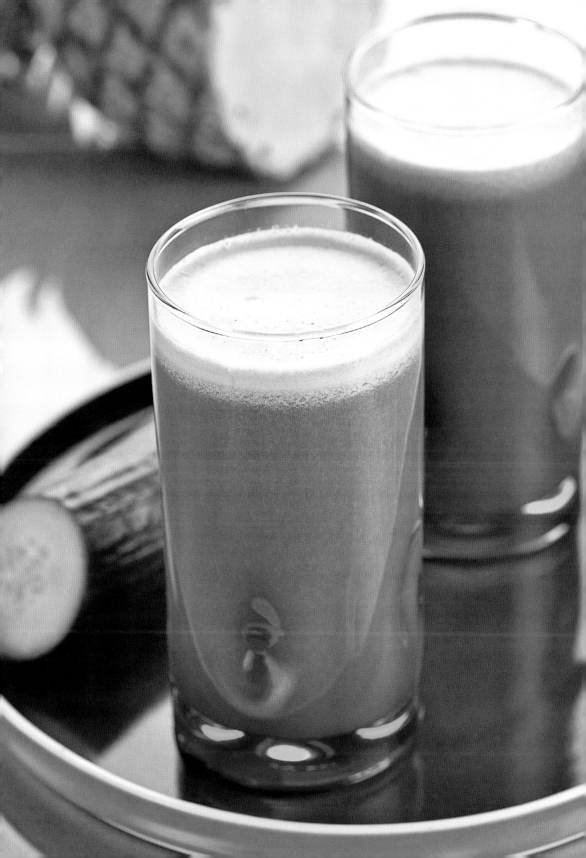

ORANGE FENNEL SPROUT >

MAKES 2 SERVINGS

2 oranges, peeled
2 stalks celery
1 bulb fennel
1 cup alfalfa sprouts

Juice oranges, celery, fennel and alfalfa sprouts. Stir.

SPRING GREEN COCKTAIL

MAKES 2 SERVINGS

8 spears asparagus
1 cucumber
1 tomato
½ lemon, peeled

Juice asparagus, cucumber, tomato and lemon. Stir.

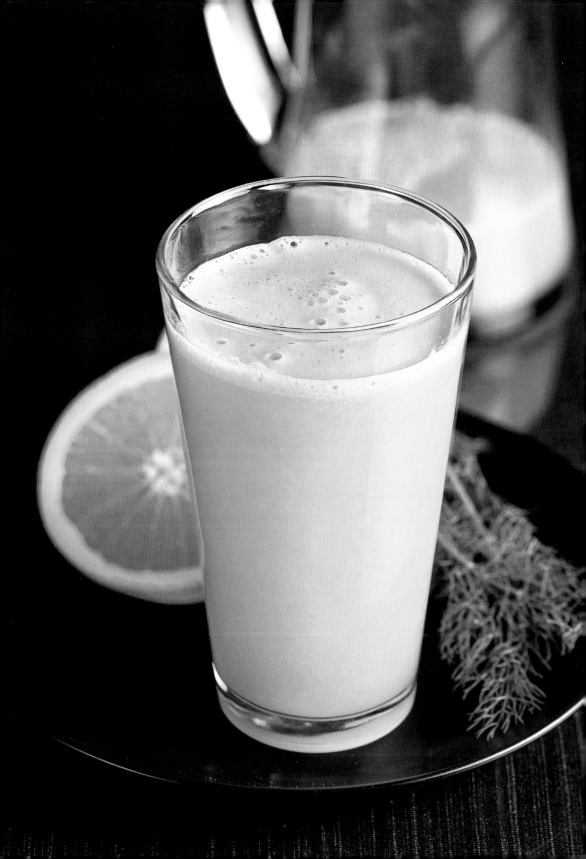

RED CABBAGE AND PINEAPPLE >
MAKES 2 SEO-RVINGS

¼ red cabbage
¼ pineapple, peeled

Juice cabbage and pineapple. Stir.

GREEN BERRY BOOSTER
MAKES 2 SERVINGS

1 cup fresh blueberries
1 cucumber
1 apple
4 leaves collard greens, Swiss chard or kale
½ lemon, peeled

Juice blueberries, cucumber, apple, collard greens and lemon.
Stir.

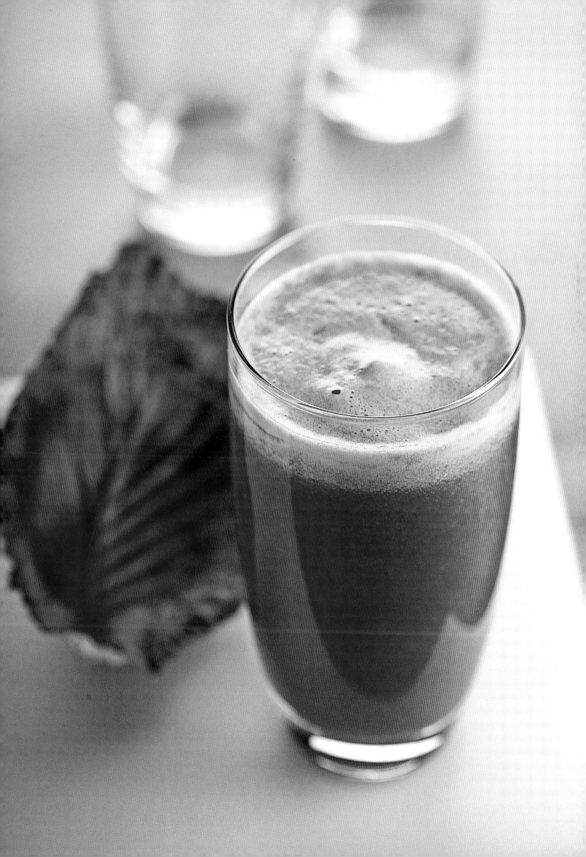

AMAZING GREEN JUICE >
MAKES 2 SERVINGS

- 1 cucumber
- 1 green apple
- 2 stalks celery
- ½ bulb fennel
- 3 leaves kale

Juice cucumber, apple, celery, fennel and kale. Stir.

AUTUMN APPLE PIE JUICE
MAKES 2 SERVINGS

- 2 apples
- ½ butternut squash, peeled
- ¼ teaspoon pumpkin pie spice

Juice apples and squash. Stir in pumpkin pie spice until well blended.

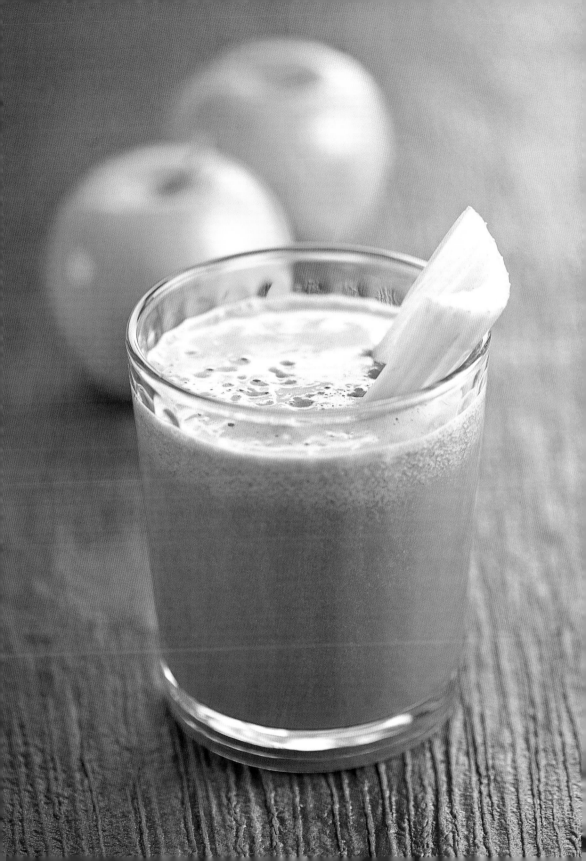

SWEET PEPPER CARROT >

MAKES 2 SERVINGS

3 carrots

1 red bell pepper

1 yellow bell pepper

Juice carrots and bell peppers. Stir.

MOJO MOJITO JUICE

MAKES 2 SERVINGS

1 cucumber

1 pear

1 cup fresh mint

½ lime, peeled

Juice cucumber, pear, mint and lime. Stir.

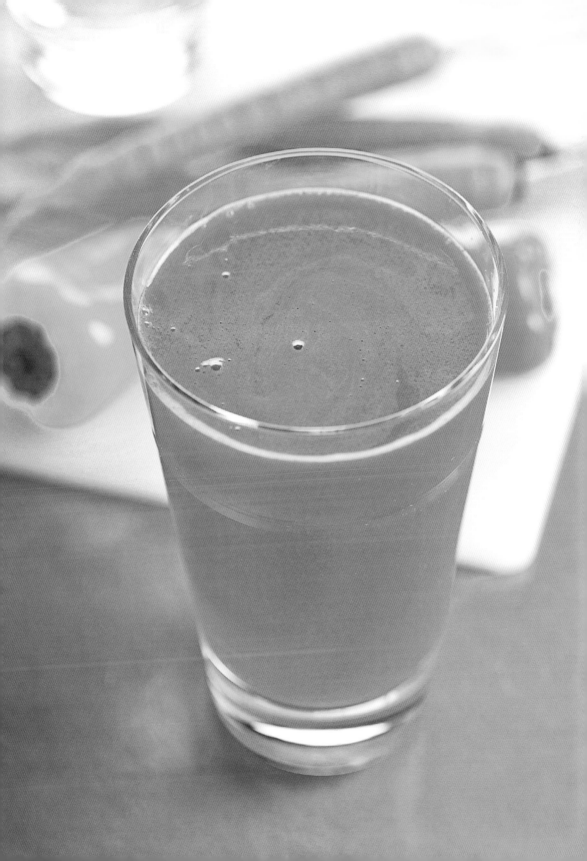

MEAN AND GREEN >

- 1 green apple
- 2 stalks celery
- 3 leaves kale
- ½ cucumber
- ½ lemon, peeled
- 1 inch fresh ginger, peeled

Juice apple, celery, kale, cucumber, lemon and ginger. Stir.

FENNEL CABBAGE JUICE

MAKES 2 SERVINGS

- 1 apple
- ¼ small green cabbage
- ½ bulb fennel
- 1 lemon, peeled

Juice apple, cabbage, fennel and lemon. Stir.

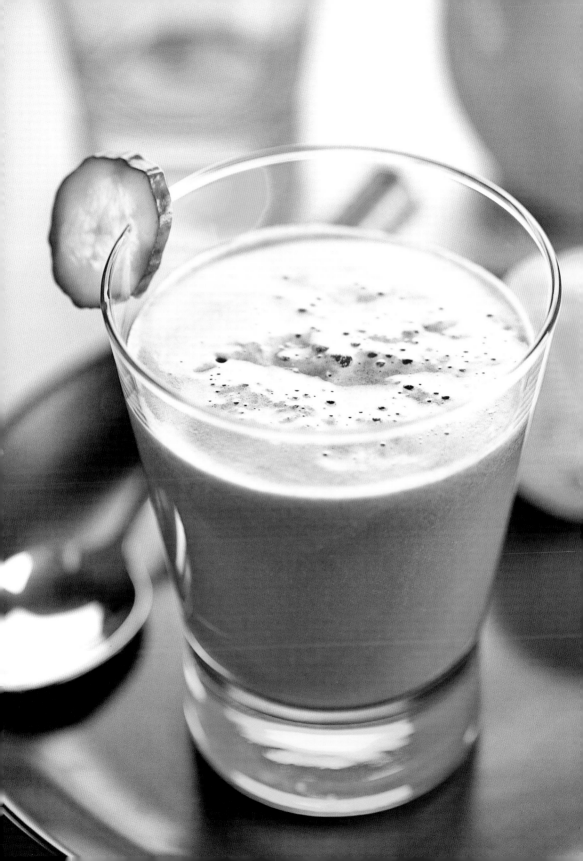

FRESH FRUIT SIPPERS

CHERRY AND MELON
MAKES 3 SERVINGS

⅛ small watermelon, rind removed

¼ cantaloupe, rind removed

¾ cup fresh cherries, pitted

Juice watermelon, cantaloupe and cherries. Stir.

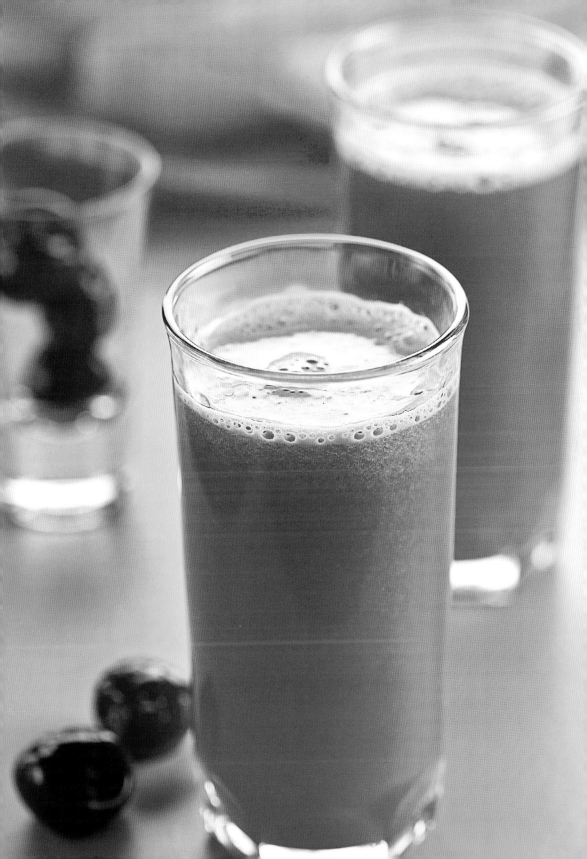

SWEET AND SPICY CITRUS >

MAKES 2 SERVINGS

5 carrots
1 orange or 2 clementines, peeled
⅓ cup fresh strawberries
1 lemon, peeled
½ inch fresh ginger, peeled

Juice carrots, orange, strawberries, lemon and ginger. Stir.

CANTALOUPE GRAPE JUICE

MAKES 2 SERVINGS

¼ cantaloupe, rind removed
¾ cup black seedless grapes
½ lemon, peeled

Juice cantaloupe, grapes and lemon. Stir.

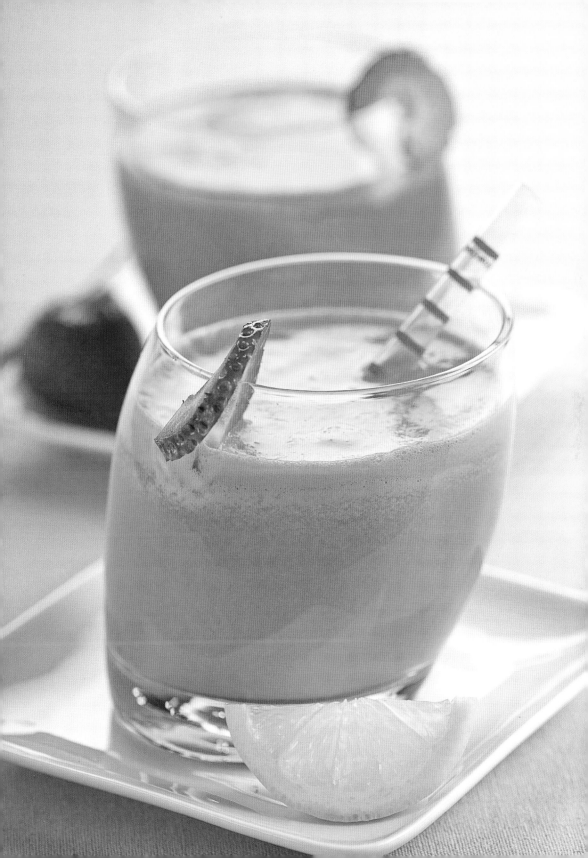

MELONADE >

¼ seedless watermelon, rind removed

1 apple

1 lemon, peeled

Juice watermelon, apple and lemon. Stir.

FANTASTIC FIVE JUICE

MAKES 2 SERVINGS

1 tangerine, peeled

½ peach

½ apple

½ pear

½ cup green seedless grapes

Juice tangerine, peach, apple, pear and grapes. Stir.

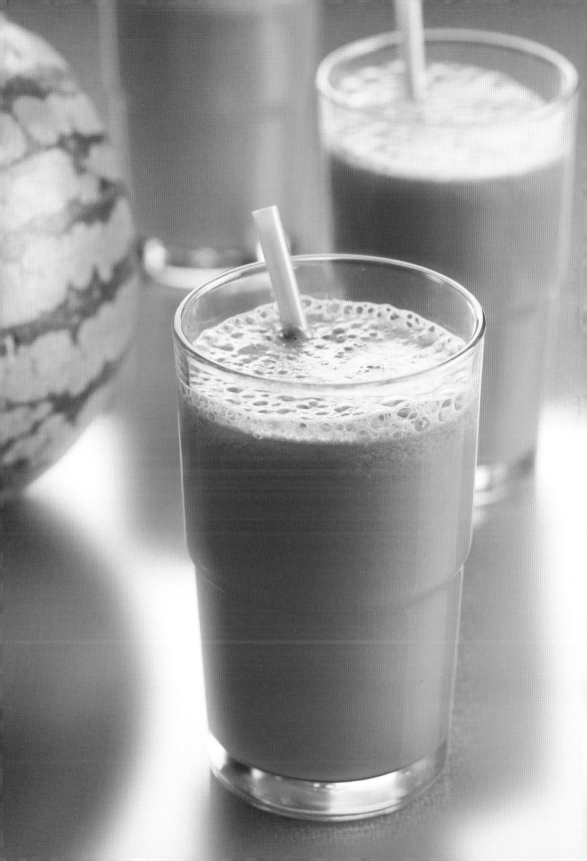

TANGERINE GINGER SIPPER >
MAKES 2 SERVINGS

1 tangerine, peeled

1 pear

¼ lemon, peeled

½ inch fresh ginger, peeled

Juice tangerine, pear, lemon and ginger. Stir.

COOL APPLE MANGO
MAKES 2 SERVINGS

1 mango, peeled

1 apple

1 cucumber

½ inch fresh ginger, peeled

Juice mango, apple, cucumber and ginger. Stir.

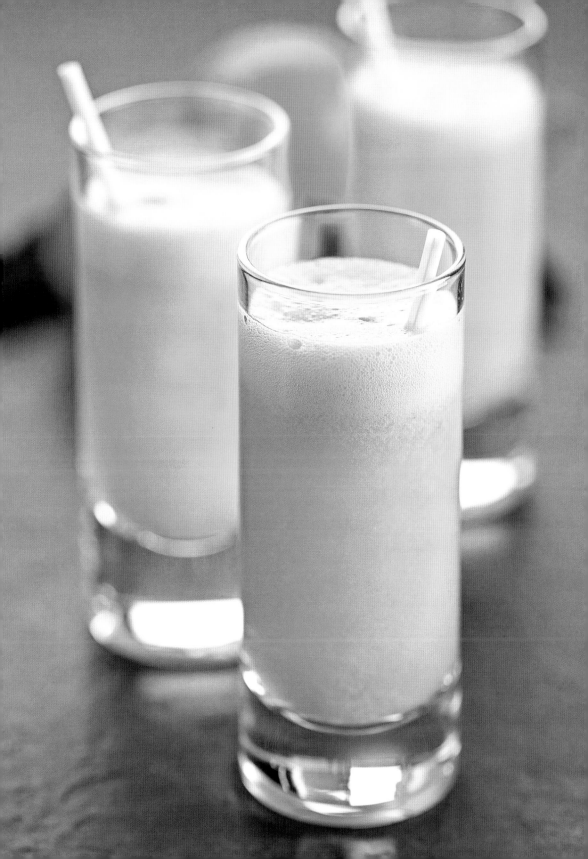

PLEASING PEAR MELON >
MAKES 3 SERVINGS

¼ honeydew melon, rind removed

1 pear

½ cucumber

Juice honeydew, pear and cucumber. Stir.

POPEYE'S FAVORITE JUICE
MAKES 1 SERVING

2 cups packed spinach

¼ pineapple, peeled

1 cup fresh raspberries

Juice spinach, pineapple and raspberries. Stir.

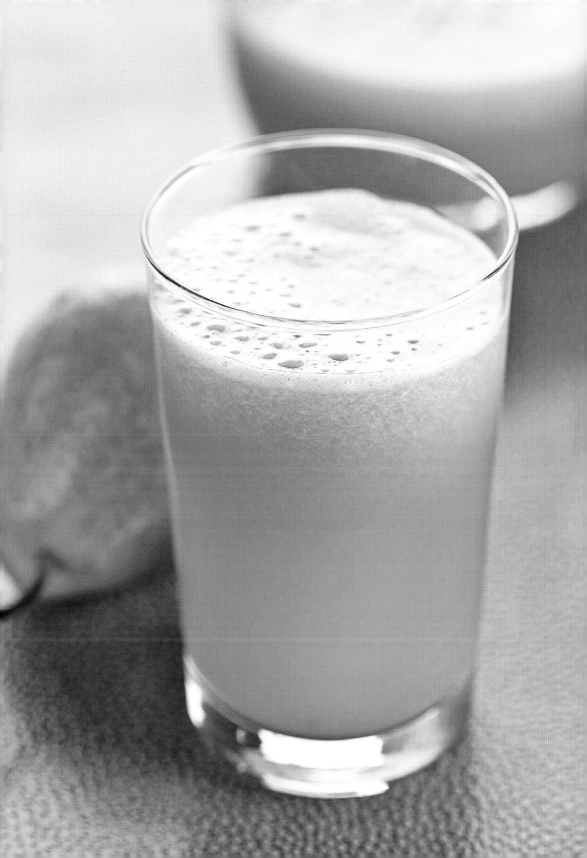

PEACHY KEEN >

MAKES 2 SERVINGS

2 peaches

1 cup red seedless grapes

¼ lemon, peeled

Juice peaches, grapes and lemon. Stir.

TROPICAL FRUIT FLING

MAKES 2 SERVINGS

¼ pineapple, peeled

1 orange, peeled

½ mango, peeled

½ cup fresh strawberries

½ cup coconut water

Juice pineapple, orange, mango and strawberries. Stir in coconut water until well blended.

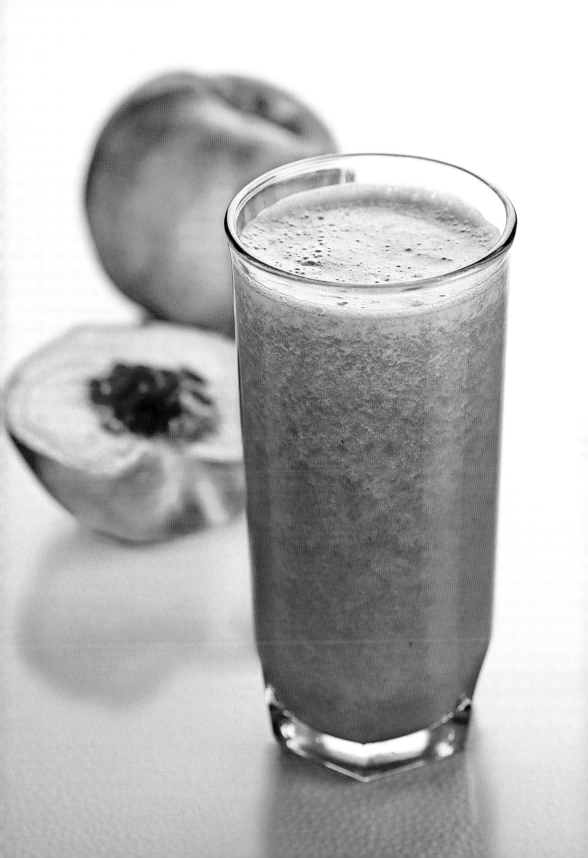

REFRESHING STRAWBERRY JUICE >

MAKES 2 SERVINGS

2 **cups fresh strawberries**

1 **cucumber**

¼ **lemon, peeled**

Juice strawberries, cucumber and lemon. Stir.

KALE MELON

MAKES 1 SERVING

4 **leaves kale**

2 **apples**

⅛ **seedless watermelon, rind removed**

¼ **lemon, peeled**

Juice kale, apples, watermelon and lemon. Stir.

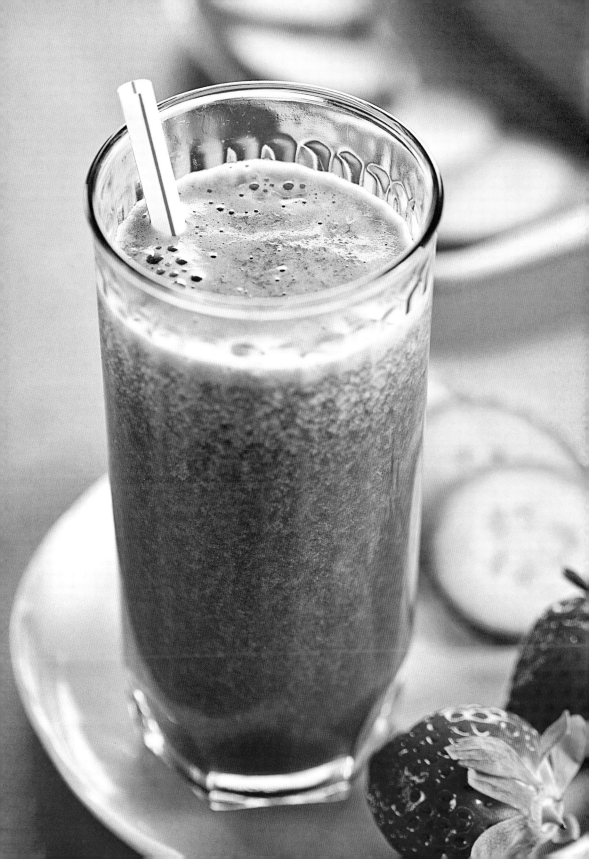

KIWI TWIST >

2 kiwis, peeled

2 pears

½ lemon, peeled

Juice kiwis, pears and lemon. Stir.

PEAR RASPBERRY

MAKES 2 SERVINGS

2 pears

1½ cups fresh raspberries

½ cucumber

Juice pears, raspberries and cucumber. Stir.

METRIC CONVERSION CHART

VOLUME MEASUREMENTS (dry)

$1/8$ teaspoon = 0.5 mL
$1/4$ teaspoon = 1 mL
$1/2$ teaspoon = 2 mL
$3/4$ teaspoon = 4 mL
1 teaspoon = 5 mL
1 tablespoon = 15 mL
2 tablespoons = 30 mL
$1/4$ cup = 60 mL
$1/3$ cup = 75 mL
$1/2$ cup = 125 mL
$2/3$ cup = 150 mL
$3/4$ cup = 175 mL
1 cup = 250 mL
2 cups = 1 pint = 500 mL
3 cups = 750 mL
4 cups = 1 quart = 1 L

VOLUME MEASUREMENTS (fluid)

1 fluid ounce (2 tablespoons) = 30 mL
4 fluid ounces ($1/2$ cup) = 125 mL
8 fluid ounces (1 cup) = 250 mL
12 fluid ounces ($1\frac{1}{2}$ cups) = 375 mL
16 fluid ounces (2 cups) = 500 mL

WEIGHTS (mass)

$1/2$ ounce = 15 g
1 ounce = 30 g
3 ounces = 90 g
4 ounces = 120 g
8 ounces = 225 g
10 ounces = 285 g
12 ounces = 360 g
16 ounces = 1 pound = 450 g

DIMENSIONS

$1/16$ inch = 2 mm
$1/8$ inch = 3 mm
$1/4$ inch = 6 mm
$1/2$ inch = 1.5 cm
$3/4$ inch = 2 cm
1 inch = 2.5 cm

OVEN TEMPERATURES

250°F = 120°C
275°F = 140°C
300°F = 150°C
325°F = 160°C
350°F = 180°C
375°F = 190°C
400°F = 200°C
425°F = 220°C
450°F = 230°C

BAKING PAN SIZES

Utensil	Size in Inches/Quarts	Metric Volume	Size in Centimeters
Baking or	$8 \times 8 \times 2$	2 L	$20 \times 20 \times 5$
Cake Pan	$9 \times 9 \times 2$	2.5 L	$23 \times 23 \times 5$
(square or	$12 \times 8 \times 2$	3 L	$30 \times 20 \times 5$
rectangular)	$13 \times 9 \times 2$	3.5 L	$33 \times 23 \times 5$
Loaf Pan	$8 \times 4 \times 3$	1.5 L	$20 \times 10 \times 7$
	$9 \times 5 \times 3$	2 L	$23 \times 13 \times 7$
Round Layer	$8 \times 1\frac{1}{2}$	1.2 L	20×4
Cake Pan	$9 \times 1\frac{1}{2}$	1.5 L	23×4
Pie Plate	$8 \times 1\frac{1}{4}$	750 mL	20×3
	$9 \times 1\frac{1}{4}$	1 L	23×3
Baking Dish	1 quart	1 L	—
or Casserole	$1\frac{1}{2}$ quart	1.5 L	—
	2 quart	2 L	—